Grandma's *Sex* Handbook

Including

Grandma's
Sex Fantasy
Cookbook

FROM:

TO:

DATE:

Message:

Audience
This book is intended to provide premarital sexual guidance to engaged couples and to improve sex for married couples. It is specifically about sex and not marriage in general. Sex is only one of many factors in making a strong marriage, but it is a very important one.

Anonymity
The names and some of the other characteristics of real people reflected in this book, including the author, have been changed to protect their identities.

Publisher
Intimate Press, USA
www.IntimatePress.com

The publisher invites your feedback, whether positive or negative, at www.GrandmasSexHandbook.com.

Dedication

This book is dedicated with extreme gratitude to those who have gone before us and were not afraid to teach their descendants about why and how to enjoy a life always blossoming with sexual fulfillment.

Sponsorship

A portion of the proceeds from the sale of each book is distributed to St. Jude Children's Research Hospital (www.stjude.org). Additional support may be provided to organizations that work to prevent or help victims of Female Genital Mutilation (FGM).

Special Appreciation To:

JC1, CJ, WF, AE, DM, RJ, JM, LO, RW, AD, JC2, JC3, KW, EN, MC, ER, JS, TM, DC, SL, NB, JL, BF, TL, KH, FD, BD, JW, BF, SW, MV, AB, TH, MS, CO, JS, SA, CC, CG, DP, DC, PM, FT, CW, CH, MH, JD, DR, SW, IL, SE, AM, DO, NC, AT, NP, RN, and EB.

First printing: February 2009

ISBN: 978-0-578-02075-4

Library of Congress Control Number: 2009926822

032-9160300-31552
001-6055819-21501
021-7560000-21502
011-7195900-08000

Grandma's Sex Handbook

Table of Contents

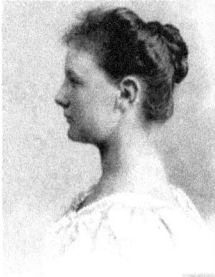

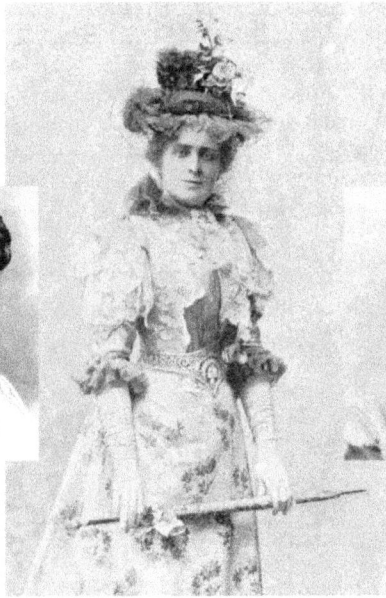

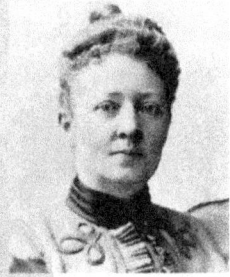

A FAMILY TRADITION OF SEX

Okay, that's supposed to be a cute chapter title. The fact is that everyone has a family tradition of sex, or none of us would be here. A more accurate title would be, and what might be somewhat unique within our family, is a tradition of very explicit sex advice being passed down through the women in our family.

As you'll see, this book isn't about the birds and the bees, that is, it's not about how babies are made, although that's mentioned briefly. It's about orgasms, mainly. How to have them, and how to make them great, for both you and your husband.

I'm Grandma Anne. That's a pseudonym I go by in this book. I am a grandmother, but just barely. The foundation of this book is based on the sex advice I got from my Grandmother "Flora", who is still alive at the age of 102! It's been our tradition to pass down sex advice from grandmother to granddaughter (or granddaughter-in-law) for at least eight generations. My Grandma got it from her Grandma, and she thinks it began well before that, but she's not sure just how far back it goes.

I didn't know anything about this tradition until I got engaged to be married and became a recipient of "the advice". And I never thought about having to pass it on until I had my first child and my Mom pointed out that it would be *her* responsibility to pass on the family sex advice to my newborn daughter when she got engaged. I would have to wait until I had grandchildren who got engaged before I could pass it on.

That got me started thinking about the responsibility I'd have someday. And I didn't like it. Actually, I was terrified. It was one thing to listen to my Grandma and repeat "Uh-huh" a million times, but it was quite another to think I would someday open my mouth and talk, out-loud, about sex. To another person. To my own granddaughter!

I honestly didn't think I could do it, but I was equally upset at the thought of breaking a multi-generation tradition. And the truth was that Grandma's advice had helped me immensely, and I certainly didn't want to deny that knowledge and understanding to my heirs. Not too long ago, this came to the forefront of my thinking when my oldest daughter gave birth to a beautiful baby girl.

Then I found out I have cancer. Nasty, life-threatening cancer. However, I discovered there's actually a side-effect to cancer that can be beneficial: soul-searching. And among many reasons I didn't want to die, the one that rose to the top of the list, was that I decided I very much wanted to pass Grandma's sex advice on to my granddaughter.

Of course, I got the idea of writing it down, so I could pass it on that way, since I wasn't expected to live more than another year or so. I had no idea how much I could get written before my time was up, but with my family gathered around and taking care of everything else, I could spend most of my remaining time working on it. I used a laptop computer, which I could use in bed... in my recliner... at the table... even in the doctors' waiting rooms when someone else carried it for me.

I kept secret what I was working on, thinking I'd figure out a way so that only my grandchildren would see what I was writing. But everyone knew that I was working on something, and everyone's curiosity was getting stronger and stronger. Still, they were a little reluctant to harass an old, sick, dying person to get me to reveal the nature of my secret project.

That started to change after a chemo-session one day, after most of the vomiting was over, and I was too exhausted to lift a hand. As usual, my mind recovered before my body, and I got very frustrated about not being able to work on my project, since time was of the essence. It was Caroline's turn to sit with me, and she perceived that frustration, and asked questions about how she could help. I broke down and cried, and ended up telling her the whole story.

Caroline offered to take dictation, and to my surprise, I took her up on it. Caroline was extremely patient during those times. Sometimes I might lie there and think for five, 10, even 15 minutes without saying anything, and then only get out a single thought or maybe two, but she never complained. During my bad times, she waited, listened, and typed for me. But during some of the better times, she started offering her own remembrances from when she heard Grandma's advice and she offered her own suggestions, which were usually very good.

As I endorsed her suggestions, she made more and more, covering everything from the organizational structure of the content to grammatical improvements. Then one day, Caroline suggested a very explicit sex tip of her own. I was wowed by it, and into the manuscript it went.

I spent days thinking about that one tip, and how it could make a difference in the lives of my grandchildren, and even their grandchildren. And I never would have thought of it. One day I told Caroline how much I appreciated that, and how I had been thinking about how it could benefit countless descendants, and after awhile, she posed another suggestion: What about asking the other women in our family for ideas?

As little as a week before, I would have hated the idea, but seeing a real possibility of leaving a powerful legacy for many generations, while facing my own mortality on a daily basis, my perspective was starting to change.

Caroline told Elizabeth about my secret, and at first she was averse to participating because of the topic, but Caroline convinced her to read what I had so far. Once Elizabeth saw that, she got excited about it, and had numerous writing suggestions, and more than a few sex tips.

The three of us started working on it together and realized that we had each heard and remembered different advice, despite having the same grandmother. This wasn't surprising in light of the fact that it had never been written down, and was usually told to different people years apart.

Working together gave a more complete recollection, and let us evaluate it based on experiences from marriages to men with a variety of personalities.

Then Grandma Flora came to visit.

Gathered around my bed we told Grandma Flora what we had been doing. We were a little worried that she might object to the idea, and then we'd be in a real quandary as to what to do. We were real excited about what appeared to be growing into a wonderful book, but we wouldn't have wanted to pursue it over her objections since it never could have happened without her original contributions. Well, she loved the idea, and that really started something!

Grandma spent the better part of a week with us going over everything she could remember, everything she learned on her own, and bringing in other women in our family, including descendants of her sisters, significantly increasing the number of people who had very valuable contributions. And that included Rachael.

Rachael had *lots* of contributions, derived from a seemingly limitless imagination, and it was she who suggested the idea Grandma's Sex Fantasy Cookbook. Before you get shocked by our Cookbook, though, please read the chapter Fantasy vs. Lust beginning on page 95.

Bringing in more women from our extended family also opened up our knowledge to issues with a wider variety of men. For instance, I never would have thought about how to have a sex life with a man with erectile dysfunction, or how to have sex with a man whose penis had been torn off by bomb shrapnel in a war.

Grandma Flora knew things about family members that neither Caroline, Elizabeth, nor I knew, such as the fact that before they became Christians, one of our relatives had been a professional prostitute, and another had been a lesbian. Most of the ladies in our extended family had many suggestions and tips, so many that we had to reorganize parts of the book to fit them all in, and the Fantasy Cookbook really did take on a collection-of-favorite-recipes feeling.

I had begun with the idea of using a one-at-a-time print-on-demand publisher, so that family members would pay for each copy and they would be printed as they were needed. But after Grandma Flora got involved, she suggested that we write it for the general public, as the information is appropriate for any Christian couple, not just our family. Especially considering how easy it is for teens to get access to online porn when they may not have a mature perspective in which to integrate it. The decision to write it for everyone necessitated more changes, including changing all the names to pseudonyms.

There are a number of reasons why we decided to use pseudonyms. The first is that there might be people who would actually hunt down and murder Grandma "Lily" if they knew who she was, just because she converted from Islam to Christianity. If people could figure out who any one of us is, they would be able to figure out who she is. That reason would be enough by itself, but for most of us, we'd be embarrassed for the public to know about our sex lives.

We'd be embarrassed, but *not* ashamed, and *not* humiliated. Shame is what people should feel when they do something they know is wrong, and humiliation is what people should feel when they've done something wrong and other people find out about it.

For most people, what is proper and improper regarding sex is an important issue, and we talk a lot about that in this book. But God created us male and female, and it was He who decided to make us capable of having orgasms, and we do not apologize for that. We believe it is a gift from God, and what a gift! So let's set the tone for the explicit nature of the rest of this book with this tribute:

Thank God for orgasms!

Have you ever
had an orgasm?

If so, have you
ever had an
orgasm and
then thanked
God for it?

If not, why not?

GRANDMA WHO?

Who are we, and why should you listen to advice about sex and marriage from our Grandma and ourselves?

Well, no one in our families who heard Grandma's sex advice before they got married has ever gotten divorced. "Past performance is no guarantee of future results," but that's not a bad record, considering we have a very large family. And Grandma's advice has been credited with saving a few marriages outside our own families as women in our family shared it with dear friends in desperate trouble. Now we wouldn't try to convince you that Grandma's advice is the only reason for that great track record, but you'd have a hard time convincing us that Grandma's advice wasn't one of the biggest reasons.

Since Grandma's advice was passed down through multiple generations, the "who" has changed a bit over time. Early on, most of our family were farmers, and the wives worked every bit as hard as the husbands, each with their own kinds of work. Then there was a period after World War II that most of the women in our families were stay-at-home moms focused on light-housekeeping and heavy child-rearing while the dads worked in factories. Lately, in addition to raising children, most of us have been working full-time jobs outside our homes, mostly in offices.

Grandma's sex advice is based on helping Christian women who really want to treat their husbands as well as they can physically and emotionally, and maximize the joy in their own lives based on relationships that are strong and healthy. While the best relationships will give equal care to spiritual and mental issues in addition to sex, this is a sex advice book, and it focuses on the physical aspect of marriage. A major goal is to help husbands and wives learn to treat each other with respect in their physical relationship, so that satisfaction and fulfillment in sex can enhance their mental and spiritual well-being. We are more than sexual objects, but sexuality is an important part of who we are.

Is there anyone Grandma's advice won't help? Yes. It won't straighten out a bent twig, as Grandma Flora says. If you're married to a guy who is inconsiderate, you won't learn anything in this book that will make him more considerate. If you're married to a guy who chases every skirt that walks by, this won't make him stop that. If you're married to a guy who abuses you physically, mentally, or emotionally, this won't turn him into a good person. And if you're only interested in what your husband can do for you, find someone else to give this book to, because Grandma's advice won't help you a bit.

If you're not a Christian, and if you're only interested in what you can do to have or give more orgasms, you may or may not find Grandma's advice worthwhile. But even if you're an atheist, you may want to try to see life a little from our perspective.

Some of our advice is presented in the form of quotes, where we thought it appropriate, so here's a cast of characters to help keep in mind who's who:

Anne: *The writer.* The primary author of this book, I worked on a college newspaper, worked for a magazine, and have had several short stories and poems published. That's all it takes to qualify as an expert in my family.

Brenda: *The low-libido but satisfied soccer mom.* Brenda is satisfied with one orgasm per month *or less*, and is very reluctant to experiment for her own satisfaction. But she's very devoted to keeping her husband totally satisfied, which means she has frequent intercourse and uses a wide variety of techniques aimed at her husband's erotic stimulation. Her primary satisfaction comes from satisfying him.

Caroline: *The quiet one.* Caroline is always there, always listening. She rarely speaks, but when she does, through her sweet, quiet voice, we're always amazed at the thoughtful things she has to say. You will be, too.

Dora: *The theologian's wife and Biblical scholar.* Dora studies Greek and Hebrew on her own, *for fun,* and her husband is a Greek and Hebrew scholar at a very conservative Protestant seminary. Being in our family, they've spent a lot of time studying what the Bible has to say about sex and sexuality, and they've vetted many of the ideas that we've come up with to see if they're consistent with Godly lives. What we've learned from them has been a major surprise to many of us, and especially the women who have married into our family who previously held very restrictive views of sex within marriage.

Elizabeth: *The bookworm and researcher.* Once we began this project, Elizabeth devoured tons of material from popular books, academic studies, and research organizations. Not satisfied with that, she did some research of her own on the traits of pornography preferred by men (pictures and video) and women (written stories). Most of us started out thinking this kind of information would be simplistic and obvious, but Elizabeth's insights were very enlightening. And stimulating.

Grandma Flora: At 102 years of age when this book began, Grandma Flora was our oldest living contributor, and a matriarch with long-term, pre-technology perspectives on sex. She was a daughter of Great-Grandma Nora, and Granddaughter of Great-Great-Grandma Theodora.

Grandma Victoria: Another of the daughters of Great-Grandma Nora, some of whose descendants also contributed to this book.

Great-Grandma Nora: Born on a farm in 1872, Nora had seven children who lived long enough to raise families of their own, and we believe she passed down the family tradition to at least thirty families of grandchildren.

Great-Great-Grandma Theodora: Born in 1844 to parents who had immigrated to the United States from Europe, our sex-advice tradition goes back at least to this matriarchal ancestor, who passed her advice directly to Grandma Flora and Grandma Victoria, among others.

Heather: *The mathematician.* E.g., Say you get married at 20, live to 70, and have an average of 2 orgasms a week for 50 years. That equals 5,200 orgasms. Increase the average orgasms per week to 2.5, and you'll experience an additional 1,300 orgasms, or an increase of 25%. Heather actually likes calculating things like this. No one else does.

Jennifer: *The psychologist.* Dr. Jennifer is a very experienced marriage counselor. In Jennifer's work, the most common problem is with poor communication between spouses, but sex is also a common issue, especially if you count poor communication about sex.

Kelly: *The former lesbian.* No lectures here about lesbianism, but for those who say there's no such thing as a former lesbian... we say you haven't met Kelly. Kelly grew up believing she was a lesbian, and lived happily as a practicing lesbian for years, but when she became a Christian, she began to have second thoughts. Over a period of years, her desires changed, she quit practicing lesbianism, eventually married a man in our family, and now states unequivocally that she's been as content with her heterosexuality as she ever was with her homosexuality. As far as our family and this collection of Grandma's sex advice, Kelly has been able to provide some unique insights into feminine eroticism. She now has 2 children and hopes to pass on Grandma's sex advice to many grandchildren.

Lily: *The former Moslem.* A Moslem until around age 30, Lily became a Christian and moved to the United States before marrying into our family. She also lived in other countries, and she was able to expand our knowledge to several other cultures.

Rachael: *The wild one.* Rachael constantly overflows with wild, imaginative ideas that the rest of us dare each other to try. Like all of us, she learned a lot from Yvette, but she quickly graduated from student to teacher. The Sex Fantasy Cookbook chapter was Rachael's superlative idea, as were many of the "recipes".

Synthia: A synthesis (get it?) of the rest of the women in our family who have provided feedback on our ideas, and suggested some of their own. This is also a "person" I sometimes quote when there's a dispute as to who said something first, or when it represents a consensus of us all.

Yvette: *The former prostitute.* Yvette was a high-end call girl trained by a very successful Madame to satisfy the fantasies of the rich and powerful. It's reliable evidence that she was very good at it since she had a small number of repeat customers who paid as much as $1000 per night for her talent. Yes, talent. As you'll learn from her contributions to this book, high-caliber sex means a lot more than lying on the bed. All that was before she became a Christian, and then a wife, married to a cousin of mine who always seems to be smiling. And yes, she now happily limits her attentions to her husband, but that doesn't mean she's forgotten any of the tricks of her former trade.

Sex Tip:

Proverbs 31:10-31 is the famous passage in the Bible that describes a wife of noble character, and Grandma Synthia urges all wives to strive for those ideals. But that describes how a wife is seen outside the bedroom, and has not a word about her conduct inside the bedroom. Grandma Synthia has her own exhortation for that realm:

Be *wild* in bed!

GRANDMA'S SEX ADVICE SUMMARY

Grandma Flora had a lot to tell me about sex. When I got engaged, she came over and spent several days giving me her advice, mostly on long walks or sitting on our front porch swing, just the two of us.

Now, telling several days worth of details about sex to someone who had never had sex could have been like pouring water into a bucket with no bottom, but Grandma was well prepared for my ignorance. She related each of the many details to two points, and she repeated those points over and over again. That had the effect of drilling them into my head well enough that I would never forget them, and it gave my mind some structure to help remember many of the details.

So to get you started, here are the two main principles of Grandma's sex advice:

1.   Enjoy sex.
2.   Keep your husband satisfied.

All the details Grandma shared with me were to explain *why* and *how*, and that's what's covered in the rest of this book. Some folks may not care about the why, but for the rest of us, many of the how's are impossible to consider without first being convinced of the why.

My Great-Great-Grandma gave the whys and how's to my Grandma, my Grandma gave them to me, and now I and my sisters, sisters-in-law, cousins, and aunts have written them for my Granddaughter, and for anyone else who wants to know.

Here are some of the key points that will be covered elsewhere in this book:

- Your vagina isn't dirty, evil, or unclean. It's part of God's *wonderful* design.

- Your clitoris isn't dirty, evil, or unclean. It's part of God's *wonderful* design.

- It's okay to enjoy sexual pleasure. In fact, there appears to be no function for the clitoris other than to provide a woman with sexual pleasure. And if you can't enjoy sex, you'll rob your husband of a critical part of *his* sex life.

- Cunnilingus is okay. It allows your husband to give you an incredible gift. Forbidding this is unfair to your husband, and does not allow him to fulfill an important aspect of his sexual life. And yes, it's in the Bible.

- Masturbation is okay. And yes, it is possible, and even easy, to masturbate without committing the sin of lust.

- Sexual fantasy is *not* the same thing as lust.

- Being sexually assertive is okay. It's not only okay, it's *required* to fully meet your duty to help your husband.

- Sexy language in the bedroom is okay. This can sometimes be a great way to boost excitement in the bedroom.

And here's one of the key Bible passages regarding sex:

> *"The husband should fulfill his marital duty to his wife, and likewise the wife to her husband. The wife's body does not belong to her alone but also to her husband. In the same way, the husband's body does not belong to him alone but also to his wife. Do not deprive each other except by mutual consent and for a time, so that you may devote yourselves to prayer. Then come together again so that Satan will not tempt you because of your lack of self-control."*[1]

---

[1] Holy Bible, NIV, 1 Corinthians 7:3-5

BEFORE MARRIAGE

Until my family and I began writing down Grandma's sex advice, it never covered advice about such things as deciding who to marry. It was advice specifically about sex, given right before marriage.

The writing process, however, eventually involved at least as much discussion as writing, and we lost count of how many times a comment included something like, "I wish I had known before I got engaged..." As a result, we decided to add this chapter to provide our collective experience and wisdom, such as it is, on these topics of great importance to women before they get engaged to be married.

First we'll talk about several aspects of having sex before marriage, and then we'll talk about the issues involved with dating and the processes that eventually lead to marriage. Here's the outline:

- Sex Before Marriage
  - The Sexual Meltdown
  - Promiscuous Sex
  - Sexual Significance
- Dating
  - Exploring
  - Matching
  - Winning Ways
  - Crashing
  - Waiting
  - Engagement & Marriage

This entire chapter is available online for free at www.GrandmasSexHandbook.com

Sex Before Marriage

Some people seem to think that having a high percentage of single people engaged in sexual activity is a recent occurrence. In the United States, especially, many people look at the reputation of the 1960's and the age of "free-love" as a point when pre-marital sex increased dramatically.

While there is some truth in that idea, it is also true that young people in love have always been tempted by sex, and there have always been large numbers of them who caved in to their carnal desires.

As part of life, these people eventually grew up and had children of their own, and when their children became old enough to get interested in the opposite sex, some of these grown-ups actually remembered the temptations they faced when they themselves were young. And some of the grown-ups occasionally considered that perhaps, just maybe, young people might still experience sexual temptations, and perhaps, just maybe, the grown-ups could help the young people avoid some of the mistakes they made when they were young.

That's the purpose of this section of advice. First for those who want to avoid sex before marriage, then for the sexually promiscuous, and finally we have some thoughts on the significance of sex to people with different perspectives.

The most common mistake for couples who want to remain virgins until their wedding night is undoubtedly what we call the *Sexual Meltdown*.

The Sexual Meltdown

A sexual meltdown is a rapid decline in self-control caused by increasingly erotic sensations that overwhelm reason and cause a complete failure of moral restraint, resulting in sexual intercourse between a couple that started out with no intention of becoming physically intimate.

Who's vulnerable to sexual meltdowns?

It sometimes happens that casual friends get some physical contact started and get into a sexual meltdown, but that's rather rare. What's extremely *common* is for two people in love with each other to get into a meltdown. A couple in love can be quite blind to real-world issues – they're usually looking at life through rose-colored glasses where only good things can happen. And engaged couples are especially vulnerable... they're already planning to get married and have sex, it's just a matter of time, so what's the big deal about a few weeks, or a few months? (We'll address that question in a minute.)

So, any two people who could possibly develop sexual feelings for each other are potentially susceptible, but the most vulnerable are the couples who are the closest emotionally.

And the most vulnerable of all? Couples who are convinced that it could never happen to them. Couples who know it could happen to them can do what it takes to avoid it; those who think it can't happen to them won't take any precautions.

What starts a sexual meltdown?

Touching. A touch that causes a sensation that is pleasurable, which makes them want more, which leads to more touching, and the touching becomes more and more intimate to keep increasing the intensity of the pleasurable feelings.

Any kind of touch can ignite a firestorm. What's meant as a simple peck-on-the-cheek kiss can linger a moment longer than intended, which leads to an embrace, a full-body hug, full-on kissing, and more. Simply holding hands can set physical passion to simmering, which can lead, perhaps subconsciously, to sitting or walking a little closer together, which leads each person to become more aware of the other's body, how close it is, and how good it feels.

This is touching that causes sexual arousal. It may seem minor at first, but it can heat up with amazing speed. The closer a couple is emotionally, the more susceptible they are. For a young couple in love, passions can come so easily and so fast, *any* kind of physical touching can spark sexual arousal.

There's a term for physical touching that causes sexual arousal: it's called *foreplay*, and it's exactly what married couples do to get their bodies and minds ready to have sexual intercourse.

Once touching initiates sexual desire, it progresses rapidly from "innocent" touching, to more and more intimate touching, and physical passion begins to overwhelm the couples' ability to reason. A complete meltdown of moral restraint results in the couple having sexual intercourse.

How long between first touch and sexual intercourse? It can be as little as mere minutes if the couple is alone and their sex drives are at peak hunger. It can be hours if at least one member of the couple has great willpower or they are not alone when the meltdown starts.

How to avoid sexual meltdowns:

If you're dating casually, the following discussion will help, but for you it won't be as urgent for you as it is for a couple in love, and it will be less urgent for a couple in love than it is for an engaged couple. For all couples, and especially for engaged couples, there are 2 simple rules that will keep you from having a sexual meltdown:

1. Don't touch each other.
2. Don't spend time alone in a place where you could be physically intimate.

We must be kidding, right? No, we're completely serious, and if *you're* serious about avoiding sex until after you're married, following these two rules is the *only* way to *ensure* your success.

Don't touch each other at all, and you can't start a sexual meltdown. Don't spend time alone together in a place where you could be intimate, and you'll be *much* less tempted to touch each other.

What if you're having a really, really, hard time waiting? Well, you've got 3 options: you can wait anyway, you can go ahead and have sex, or get married right away. If you're engaged and already have a wedding date, you can move up the date.

Change your wedding date?! Are we crazy? Well, those 3 options are your only alternatives. Wait, have sex now, or get married sooner. Yes, choosing to get married sooner might mess up your extremely elaborate wedding plans. But if you don't get married sooner, you're down to 2 options. If you do start to move up the date, you'll have to tell friends and family that you're getting married sooner. They'll ask why. You'll say it's because "we just don't want to wait."[2] Everyone who's already married will know exactly what that means. And the ones who remember their own courtship will sympathize with you. Oh, you could also tell them it's to save money – that sounds a lot less like you're about to rip each other's clothes off.

If you decide to wait, **it's not hard to wait for sex if you don't touch each other and don't spend time alone where you could be physically intimate**. Yes, you want to touch each other, and yes, you want to be physically intimate. But if you have *an even stronger desire to wait* until your wedding night, then keep plenty of other people around you whenever you're together. No, that doesn't mean someone else is in the living room while you and your lover are necking in the den. Sorry, you have to be in the same room with your escorts or it won't help. If you're engaged, don't spend time alone together or you'll be drawn together like two irresistible magnets.

If, wherever you are, you suddenly discover that everyone else left and the two of you are now alone, one of you run away. Seriously. Unless you secretly want to go ahead and have sex and pretend it was an accident, one of you leave *immediately*.

There's one other technique that has helped some people who are casually dating. By casually dating, we mean couples with little or no interest in a physical relationship, at least not in the current stage of their relationship. For people dating casually, masturbation can periodically reduce their sexual urges, and that can help avoid a sexual meltdown on casual dates where emotional levels are relatively low. Is masturbation okay? We've got a whole chapter on that coming up.

For a couple in love, and for engaged couples, periodically masturbating alone to lower the desire for sex while you're together *might* be of some help, but don't count on it. With the strong hormone levels of teens and young adults, a young person can get sexually recharged *very* quickly, so it would be unwise to depend on that.

Not allowing yourselves to touch each other and not allowing yourselves to be alone together are the best techniques if you really want to succeed in preserving your virginity until your wedding night.

---

[2] Holy Bible, NIV, 1 Corinthians 7:9 "... if they cannot control themselves, they should marry..."

Why avoid sexual meltdowns?

God says to have sex only with your spouse. That means you'll only have sex after you're married and only with that one person. And if both spouses do that, it means you'll both avoid sexually transmitted diseases and pregnancy out of wedlock. It also means you'll be obeying God.

Isn't the week before marriage close enough?

The first time you have sexual intercourse, it will probably feel amazingly-fantastically wonderful. If your first sexual experience is before marriage, it may feel just as good physically as it would if you waited until your wedding night, but that good *physical* feeling will be offset by lots of *emotional* negatives such as disappointment, disillusionment, regret, shame, etc. If your first sexual experience is on your wedding night, it will be untainted by emotional wounds. On the contrary, your success in waiting for your wedding night will magnify the physical pleasures and emotional intimacy!

Promiscuous Sex

Sexual promiscuity means a person has sex with more than one person, and includes those who have sex indiscriminately with many partners.

The most common occasion for teenagers to experience intentional sex or a sexual meltdown is after school, before the parents get home, when both parents work, or if one parent is at work and the other is not home for other reasons. This is a compelling reason for parents to do everything possible to avoid making your teenage children part-time orphans during the after-school hours.

Sex, Sexually Transmitted Diseases, and Lies

A promiscuous boy wants to have sex with a new girl. A promiscuous girl wants to have sex with a new boy. What they want is to have sex. What they don't want is to waste time talking, especially if that talking makes it less likely that they will have sex. Talking as in "By the way, I have an STD." Or "I don't love you, I just want to use your body to satisfy my body." Or talking as in having to answer, "Do you have any STD's?" It doesn't take a genius to figure out that a guy won't get much sex with: "By the way, I have an STD. Now how about taking your pants off?"

Because a promiscuous person wants to have sex, they have a very compelling, urgent desire to avoid talking about STD's, and if their partner brings it up, they tend to want to lie about it so they can hurry up and get in the other person's pants.

Maybe they don't know if they have an STD. That could be because they haven't been tested. On purpose. Because if they don't hear a doctor say they have one, they don't have to lie to say they don't know.

However, **any person who has ever has sex with one or more other people who were not virgins may have a sexually transmitted disease**. Even if they were just tested for all known STD's and they haven't had sex since. First, they may have an STD and the test had a false-negative. Second, they may have an STD that no test exists for. Third, they may have an STD that no one even knows exists yet. For example, HIV (and AIDS) was spreading rampantly for years before the medical community found it, and it took additional time to develop tests for it. Of course, they're still working hard to try to come up with a cure for it, and in the meantime, although the death rate has slowed, people still die from it.

Claims by lovers to be disease free are worthless if they have had sex with anyone since they were tested for every known STD, if they weren't tested for every known STD, if any negative result was false, or if they have any unknown or un-testable STDs. Obviously, a claim by a lover to be disease-free is also worthless if they're a liar or ignorant of the facts.

For girls especially, if a man thinks you'll have sex with him if you think he's disease-free, you're giving him a very powerful incentive to say he is disease-free whether he is or not. Many men will glibly lie in order to get in your pants if the only risk is to you. If they're already infected, they're no longer at risk. Do you think that if they love you they'll be truthful with you? If they really love you, they wouldn't take a chance of infecting you.

Gardasil STD Vaccine

Gardasil® is a vaccine against a set of sexually transmitted human papillomaviruses (HPV), which can cause some cervical, vulvar, vaginal, penile, and anal cancers. It's only effective in preventing HPV infections (and the cancers they cause), it will not help anyone already infected, and it does not work immediately. Because HPV is spread by sexual contact, it is not possible to acquire HPV if a husband and wife never have sex with anyone but each other. If, however, you are a virgin marrying someone who is not a virgin, you should get the Gardasil vaccination shots (several shots, spread several days apart) at least a month before you have sex for the first time. **If you get infected first, it's too late.**

Grandma's Sexual Promiscuity Rules

Okay, you know Grandma says it best to wait until marriage to have sex, and that she knows a lot of teens and young adults are going to have sex with multiple partners over time despite the risks and disadvantages. So our list of rules covers both possibilities:

- Don't have sex before marriage.
- If you do have sex before marriage, don't get pregnant or get a disease.
- If you do get pregnant, have the baby and give it up for adoption.
- If you do get a disease, you are morally required to tell your fiancée *before* you get married and *before* you have sex with them.

If you're promiscuous, you're very likely to become pregnant sooner or later, so here's Grandma Synthia's position on abortion and related issues. Yes, a woman has a right to control her own body. Other than rape, everything she does to get pregnant is controlling her own body. However, once she is pregnant, the embryo/fetus/baby is *inside* the mother's body, and is completely *dependent* on the mother's body, but **a baby is not part of the mother's body** because the DNA of the baby's cells are not the same as the mother's. You still demand a choice? Okay... choose life.

Sexual Significance

How spiritual a person is has a major impact on their perspective on the act of sex. At one extreme, an atheist may regard sex as nothing more than a physical act with no significance other than satisfying a physical hunger. On the other extreme, a very spiritual person may regard sex as primarily a sacred act that only incidentally happens to occur in the physical realm. In the center is a balanced position that regards sex as a natural act that includes a spiritual aspect.

The significance that a person attaches to sex influences, and may even control, many of their actions in life: who they're attracted to, who they marry, whether or not they have sex without marriage, their reaction to rape (such as anger or denial), etc.

The significance that a man and woman each attach to sex also has an impact on their suitability as spouses. A man and woman with attitudes at opposite extremes are the least compatible, and this can be a major factor in the early success or failure of a marriage.

> **Grandma Jennifer:** *The significance that a person attaches to sex may change over time, and if the marriage of a couple who are far apart in their perspectives can survive long enough, their perspectives may move closer to each other. Most commonly, a promiscuous person who regards sex primarily as a physical act, and a virgin who regards sex primarily as a spiritual act may both come to regard sex as much more of a natural act. The experience of the promiscuous may lead one to feel jaded that they missed something valuable in their limited perspective. Similarly, when a heavily spiritual person has sex with a spouse on a regular basis, and perhaps has children, the mundaneness of married sex may lead them to feel that they overestimated the spiritual aspect of sex.*

Dating

Who are you going to marry?

Dreams about Prince Charming eventually fade away, to be replaced with day-dreams about that muscular boy on the football team or that really cute guy at Church. And eventually, we get interested in one boy seriously enough to consider marriage.

In modern America, school, Church, and similar group events are common ways for boys and girls to get familiar with a wide range of people of the opposite sex, allowing them to explore among all the eligible marriage candidates.

When such exploration results in a boy and girl being attracted enough to each other to want to consider more than a casual relationship, dating is the most common social method that allows them the opportunity to get to know one another better, which in turn allows them to determine how well they really match each other.

Many teens spend years going through the process of exploring and matching without having a clue what they're doing, what kind of result their efforts may lead them to, or even why they're doing what they're doing. The most clueless just drift along with the social currents, without a goal or a care.

At the other end of the spectrum are the teens who know they want to get married, know when they want to get married, and know the kind of person they want to marry. For them, dating has a very specific goal. These folks may date some of their directionless cohorts and struggle to realize that not everyone is as focused on long-term relationship issues as they are.

Most teens are somewhere in between these two extremes, and float back and forth over time. Sometimes one will get serious about a possible a mate, and other times they'll go on dates "just for fun" as a couple or in groups, though for most, even "fun" dates have at least a little spouse-hunting interest buried in there somewhere.

So all social occasions let people explore for potential mates, and dating is a social process that allows tentative couples to apply very informal evaluations to match their interests, to find the ones who are most appealing, narrowing the field until each finds "the one".

Dating is not the only option, however. Some cultures practice arranged marriages, in which the parents do the exploring and matching, but this is rare in the United States, and parents cannot legally force marriages on their children here.

Another option, although its relatively uncommon in the U.S. today, is courtship. This is usually a more formal process than dating, and closely involves the parents in the efforts of exploring and matching.

We might point out that today, the term "dating" is also used to refer to a long-term boy-girl relationship that acts as a substitute for marriage. In this kind of relationship, the boy and girl are having sex just as they would as if they were married, and often even live together. The biggest differences between this relationship and marriage is just the lack of a ceremony and the legal rights of marriage. This is not the kind of dating we're talking about in this book.

For many young Americans today, the process of exploring and matching is so informal, they don't even realize they're doing it. Unfortunately, that also means they often do a bad job of it, which leads to many heart-rending breakups.

By paying at least a little attention to the issues covered in this chapter, a young woman or man may be able to be a little more careful in deciding who to date and what becomes of it. It may, for example, help you avoid a *Sexual Meltdown* (discussed in the previous section on Sex Before Marriage). Some of the ideas here may help improve your ability to prevent your emotional and physical passions from overwhelming the equally important mental and spiritual considerations when seeking a mate.

Exploring

When you're exploring for a potential husband among all the men in your communities and circles of friends, keep your field of vision wide. The most outgoing men get the most attention, but there are many other men who are more reserved and harder to spot.

Which kinds of men are more appropriate for you? Well, which kinds of men are you attracted to emotionally, physically, and spiritually? Which kinds of men seem to be attracted to you, and *why*? Don't focus on which men might be good lovers, focus on which men might be your best friends, because a good friend will be a great lover, but a good lover may never be a good friend. Likewise, true love will include physical desire, but mere lust will not include intimate friendship.

Another word of warning for while you're going on group outings and "fun dates": be aware that flirting can be very harmful to yourself or to the boy you flirt with. By flirting we mean teasing in a manner likely to stir up sexual desire. Laugh and joke all you want in a non-sexual way, but stay completely away from sexual innuendos.

For a man, leading him to think you're interested in him sexually, only for him to eventually realize the truth that you have no intention of having sex with him, can crush his spirit in a very painful and demeaning way. A vengeful or brutish man may go so far as to look for an opportunity to force you to have sex thinking that you owe it to him or that you deserve punishment. For you, men that you might truly like to pursue may have no interest in you when they see you flirting with another man, even if they know you're flirting with them insincerely. Or perhaps especially if they know you're flirting with someone insincerely. In addition, if you get in a habit of flirting with men, you may eventually find yourself becoming more serious about following up with a man physically if he responds to your flirtations.

So, keep your exploring clean and light. **Look for men who can be good friends.** When you find some good friends, then you're ready to start some serious matching efforts to see if one of them has the potential to become your *best* friend.

Matching

Matching is the process where you compare a potential spouse with yourself to try to determine just how compatible you are with each other. It can be methodical or haphazard, conscious or subconscious, but the more attention you give it, the more likely you are to avoid a breakup later on when you finally discover some serious incompatibilities.

You want someone to love you for who you are. But do *you* know who you are? If you're starting to fall in love with a man, do you know if he wants to have children? Do you know if you do? If you're starting to fall in love and you've always had a strong desire to have children and you learn the man you're interested in is determined never to have children, or isn't able to father children, you'll either have to forsake him or forsake your desire for children.

This is the time for Grandma to tell you: Don't try to change yourself for a man. If your character and desires don't match a man without changing yourself, you don't match each other. No matter how hard it may seem, no matter how painful, no matter how many dreams you've already invested in him... he's the wrong man. Get over him. He's the wrong man. Don't change yourself. Get over the wrong man and start looking for the right man.

How do you know if you and a particular man are a match for each other? You don't have to share the same characteristics, but the most important characteristics should at least be compatible. If you want 3 children and he wants 4, is that something one of you is willing to compromise on? It may not seem like as big a deal as one wanting children while the other is opposed to any children, and for most couples, a decision whether you might have 3 or 4 children might be put off if you both agree to see how things "work out." And if just one of you is willing to compromise on the number, then that can work out. But if both of you are unwilling to compromise on the number of children, and your numbers don't match, then that's a very bad mismatch. And it may reflect an even bigger mismatch if you are both determined to make the other person compromise.

There are many characteristics that can be matched other than those we list next, but these are some of the minimum characteristics you should consider:

Love Languages[3]
This may be the least familiar issue to you, but it may be the most important. There are 5 ways in which men and women show their love for another person, and the way in which they show love is also how they naturally expect others to show their love. They are:

1. Words of affirmation
2. Physical touch
3. Physical gifts
4. Quality time
5. Acts of service

Take a questionnaire[4] to find out what your love language is, and what your potential spouse's love language is. If your love language is physical touch, but your guy's love language is acts of service, how satisfying will your marriage be to you if you rarely get the hugs you crave? How satisfied will he be when he doesn't see you showing your love for him by doing things for him?

There are many combinations of love language strengths that are highly compatible, but there are just as many that are incompatible, and the incompatibilities can be HUGE.

---

[3] Dr. Gary Chapman, Northfield Publishing, Chicago, The Five Love Languages: How to Express Heartfelt Commitment to Your Mate (1995)
[4] http://www.fivelovelanguages.com/30sec.html

Age

For some folks, age is nearly irrelevant, but for others, it's a big deal. Have you been truthful with each other about your ages?

Character

Are you compatible in issues of honesty, diligence, and how considerate you are of others? For example, does one of you think it's okay to lie on your tax return while the other thinks it's always wrong? If the person you're considering marrying is not considerate of others, don't expect that person to give you many orgasms. Can you live with that? Can you thrive with that?

Communicativeness

How openly do you share your feelings and thoughts with each other? If one of you is talkative and the other isn't, will you both find that acceptable for the next 20 years? Is one of you so talkative it's hard for the other to get a word in edge-wise? In five years, is that going to be endearing or driving the other crazy?

Desire for Children

Do you both want children? Do you both want the same number? Are you both willing to play-it-by-ear and see how well your contraceptive methods work?

Employment plans

Do you each know the other's career plans? Do you know what the options are if things go badly in a career? Can you really commit to the worse part in "for better and for worse"?

Personality

Are you compatible in your outlook on life, in your friendliness, stability, open-mindedness, and willingness to compromise? For example, do you like to attend and host parties while your intended strongly prefers to just have quiet nights at home?

Physical attractiveness

Physical appeal isn't everything, but it's something. Do each of you like the way the other looks now? Does one of you look the way you do because you've been working very hard to keep the weight off? If so, what happens when they stop working at it quite so hard and the weight comes rushing back?

Political views

Some couples get along with very different political beliefs, but for most couples political differences are a constant source of tension. Politics can be different and yet compatible, or they can be a nail in a relationship's coffin.

Religion

Ditto on the comments for political differences. Some couples get along with very different religious beliefs, but for most couples religious differences are a constant source of tension. Have you discussed this? In detail?

Sexual diseases

Does one of you have a sexual disease that the other doesn't? Are you willing to get what the other has? Because if you get married, you will almost certainly get each other's STD's.

Views on contraception

Does either of you hold the views of the Catholic Church while the other doesn't? Once you have as many children as you want, does the man want the woman to get her tubes tied instead of him getting a vasectomy when vasectomies are so much safer?

Winning Ways

Okay, what if you think you've found the perfect match for you, but he doesn't seem to be coming around. What should you do?

Be yourself. Smile. Encourage him. Be kind to him. Consider asking him straight-out what he thinks about marrying you. Consider asking him to marry you. And if you learn with difficulty that he's not the right man for you, do your best to deal with the pain head-on.

Let Grandma assure you that you should never try to *catch* a man. Don't try to pretend to be someone you're not or behave in a way you think he'd like if that isn't really like you. Don't try to seduce a man into sex in the hopes he will then ask you to marry him. Don't try to get pregnant in the hope that he'll ask you to marry him. Don't try to beg, guilt, shame, needle, or nag him into marriage. Why not? Because if you succeed, you'll regret it. If you have to do these kinds of things to get him, *he's the wrong guy for you.*

Crashing

You were in love, and now you're not. Or you're still in love, but the man you love has turned his heart away from you. Or you're still in love and the man you love is still in love with you, but you now know that you are not right for each other. In every case, your heart may ache beyond what you think you can endure.

Don't compromise. Don't settle. Don't marry too soon just to get married. Do what you know is right, no matter how hard it is. Because no matter how hard it is to do right, it is not as hard and not as painful as doing the wrong thing.

Cry all you want. Cry all you need. But a better day is coming for you. Days so full of joy they really will make the pain you feel today fade into a distant memory. When you are up to it, start exploring again, then start matching again. The right person is out there for you. You *can* make it. You *will* make it.

Waiting

You may not be surprised that many women become very eager to get married and that their eagerness for marriage drives their emotions in most of their interactions with eligible men. You might be surprised that the same is true of many young men.

Many young people struggle for years and years with a very strong desire to get married, while they haven't found the right person yet. Perhaps that won't happen to you, but you shouldn't be surprised if it does. It's hard, and it's painful, but no matter how hard it is, it is worth it to wait for the right person and the right time.

How can you wait to get married to the right person? How can you act casual when your heart is desperate?

First of all, pray. A lot. Don't underestimate the power of pouring your heart out to God for help.

Next, keep busy with pursuing your education and a career, and with volunteer work. The busier you are, the less you'll focus on your desire for companionship with the opposite sex.

While your sex drive is still dormant, do your best to keep it that way, and keep busy. If you've started masturbating, it's okay to keep doing so, as it can periodically reduce your physical desires and make it much easier to cope with your emotional desires.

Once you are engaged, avoid being alone with your fiancée, because that's when the temptation of premarital sex will be strongest. If you've been masturbating, it's a good idea to keep doing so to keep your physical desires from becoming overwhelming when you're together.

Engagement & Marriage

You explored. He explored. You found each other. You match each other. You match *great*. He proposed. You accepted. Or you proposed and he accepted. Now, you're engaged to be married!

Hooray! Now you can read the rest of this book, get married, and start having lots and lots of sex!

Errrk... hold on a minute, there are still a few other issues to consider. Your engagement may last longer than a few hours providing many opportunities to fall into pre-marital sex, you and your fiancée need some seasoned counseling, and wedding plans can take on a life of their own. And if you've successfully avoided having sex until now, good for you... no, *great* for you, but you're not out of danger yet.

Temptations

Your engagement period may present you with your greatest sexual temptations yet, so if you haven't read the earlier section discussing *sexual meltdowns*, do it now. It starts on page 14.

Counseling

Next, let's cover counseling. Counseling isn't just for people with problems. It's also to help people avoid problems. What, you'd rather have problems?

You need to find a person or a couple with a lot of experience in counseling engaged couples. Big Churches are good places to inquire. If they don't have trained pre-marriage counselors on staff, they should at least know some they can refer you to.

Most couples don't think they need counseling before they experience pre-marriage counseling. And half of those couples will contribute to the 50% divorce rate in this country.

How can counseling help? It can provide a structured setting with an impartial 3rd party to help you and your beloved review critical issues and decisions. For example, they can go over issues of compatibility and make sure you haven't missed any big issues or glossed them over.

They can help you reach a deeper level of understanding of a covenant-level commitment to marriage. For instance, when you get married, you could each sign an irrevocable, unlimited power-of-attorney for each other. Do you realize what that would mean if one of you decided to leave the other? Would you still agree to get married if such a document could permanently ruin your ability to free yourself financially from your spouse even if you got divorced? Hmm?

A good counselor can help you consider financial issues that you've never thought about... issues that could cause serious disagreements in the future if not planned for now.

You can read Grandma's Sex Handbook cover to cover, but a counseling plan can make sure you and your groom actually discuss each important area of sexuality, so that you don't have any nasty surprises or disappointments after you're already married.

Kegel Exercise

Did you know your vagina is very muscular? Did you know you can exercise those muscles? And that if you do, you can improve your own orgasms and make sex more fun for your husband?

It can be difficult to learn how to control a muscle you've never consciously controlled before, but the easiest way to exercise your vaginal muscles is to try to squeeze them while you're peeing, so you stop the flow of urine. Yes, it takes some getting used to, but it becomes easy after that. And it's *really* worth it!

Scheduling Your Honeymoon

Read the honeymoon section of the Great Sex chapter for lots of ideas regarding what happens on your honeymoon. Here, we'll just give you one word of advice about planning for your honeymoon: Estimate your menstruation schedule as well as you can, and try to plan your wedding (the start of your honeymoon) in between your periods. The farther out you set your wedding date, the less accurate your estimate will be. Even if you've been very regular, the stresses of preparing for your wedding may cause some changes.

If it doesn't work out and you're on your period on your wedding night, it's okay, it won't ruin it if you don't let it.

If you've chosen a considerate husband, he may be bothered by it far less than you. Some new husbands, especially the more intellectual ones, may be fascinated by the opportunity to learn about your periods first hand. He may want to try to experience it with you as much as possible. If so, let him, for his sake, even if you think your periods are really gross. It may be annoying as all get-out to you, but to him, it may be new and interesting. Especially if he had no sisters to pick up snippets of info from.

While you're scheduling your wedding and honeymoon, you should consider scheduling an appointment with a gynecologist, a doctor who specializes in the female reproductive system, to have her/him examine your hymen. Your hymen may already be broken, and if not, most hymens break easily when you have intercourse for the first time. However, some women have extremely thick hymens, and breaking them can be difficult and very painful. Your gynecologist can check that, and if needful, can give you a local anesthetic and cut it for you.

Oh, and there's one other thing you should do before your honeymoon...
finish reading Grandma's Sex Handbook!

Your Wedding

Okay, whether you've been planning your wedding for years or not, it won't hurt to listen to a little advice, perhaps a little *reasonable* advice.

There's no such thing as a perfect wedding. Plan all you want, as long as you're enjoying it, but expect that something will go wrong on your wedding day.

If you build all your emotions around an expectation of a perfect ceremony and a perfect day, then when something goes wrong, you've set yourself up for your wedding day to be "ruined." In such cases, there's often anger and crying in place of joy, and you may set off for your honeymoon in an attitude of disappointment.

If instead you build all your emotions around the beginning of your marriage, then a few things can go wrong without ruining anything. In this case, everyone roles with the punches, enjoys the celebration of your union, and you set off for your wedding night in good spirits.

Now please bear with an old Grandma while she pleads a case for restraint:

Weddings don't *have* to be expensive. What's the difference between $100 worth of flowers and $10,000 worth of flowers? A lot of flowers, yes. But is this your *flower* day? Is it your *12-bridesmaids* day? Is it your *wedding reception* day? Or perhaps, could it be the day you marry the man you love? If the latter, are some extra flowers so important?

Yes, your wedding is an important date. Yes, it should be memorable. Your wedding photo album will be exciting... at first. And it may stay out on your coffee table for a long time. Even years. But it won't be looked at very often. You'll be too busy with life and building new memories. And eventually, it will be put on a shelf. It may come off the shelf a few times over the years, but rarely. So here's a question: how precious is a memory if the only way you can remember it is to see it in a photo album? Here's a suggestion: Let the most precious memories from your wedding be those you don't need a photo of in order to remember. And the things that make precious memories are not things you purchase.

Oh, my darling,
and oh, the delight
of my eyes!

Basic Sex

Most readers will be given this book a few weeks before your marriage, which is the best time to start seriously studying sex if you're waiting until marriage before you have sex.

In this chapter on basic sex, we'll study the plumbing, first yours, then your husband's. Then we'll talk about what kinds of sex there are, sexual positions, and issues regarding pregnancy, since that's often the result of basic sex.

- The Female World
  - Female Anatomy
  - The Female Reproductive Cycle
  - Female Erogenous Zones
  - Female Sexual Response Cycle
- The Male World
  - Male Anatomy
  - Male Erogenous Zones
  - Male Sexual Response Cycle
- Types Of Sex
  - Teasing / Flirting
  - Foreplay / Petting
  - Manual Sex
  - Oral Sex
  - Vaginal Intercourse
  - Anal Intercourse
  - Other Forms Of Sex
- Sex Positions
- Pregnancy
  - Getting Pregnant
  - Contraception
  - Unplanned Pregnancy
  - Abortion

The Female World

Female Anatomy

You need to know what your sex parts are and how they work to get the most out of them. Figures 1 and 2 show your reproductive and other pelvic organs, and Figures 3 and 4 show a woman's genitals. This is one advantage of a book over Grandma's verbal descriptions.

Your genitals may be hard to see without a mirror, so if you haven't looked carefully before, take a hand-held mirror and this book into your bathroom, if your bathroom has a strong light, and find all the parts you can reach. Your clitoris will be the most sensitive to touch. It varies in size a little bit between women, but for most women, when you're not sexually aroused, it will be a little bump. When you become sexually aroused, it gets a little bigger.

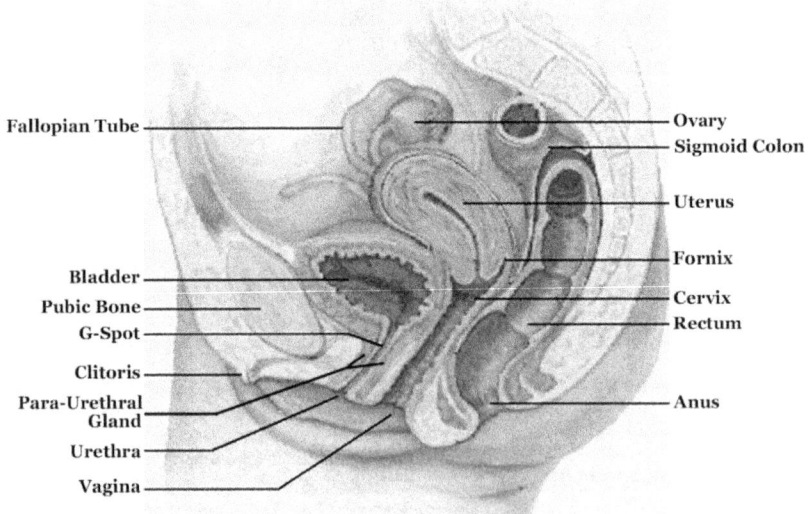

Figure 1. Cross-Sectional View of Female Pelvic Organs

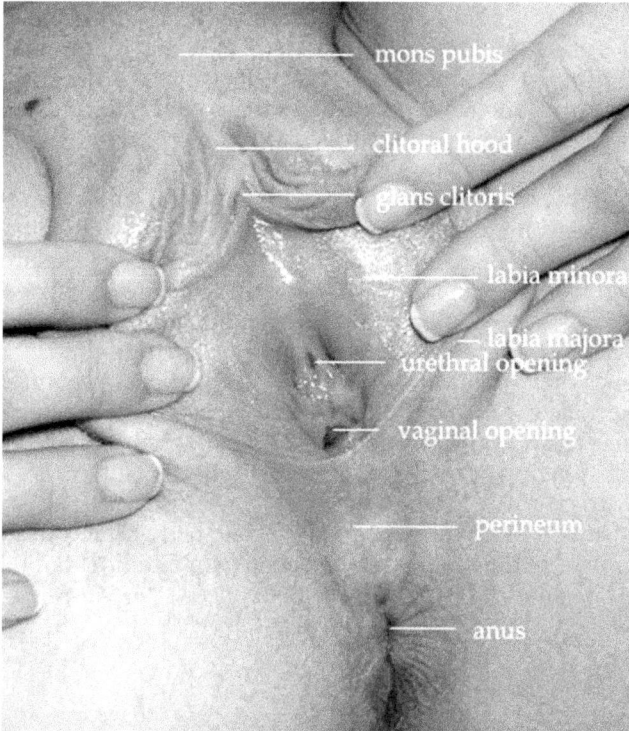

Figure 2. Photo of Female External Genitalia

It's important for you to at least be familiar with your sexual body parts. The photo in Figure 2 is included because it can be very difficult for some women to find some of their anatomical parts based on drawings alone, and this photo is very clear.

What are the most important parts of your body regarding sex? The **clitoris** is the most important for most women to reach on orgasm. The **vagina** is the most important part of your body for vaginal intercourse, obviously.

However, your genitalia are not the only parts of your body that are important for sex, and we'll cover that more in a section coming up on female erogenous zones. For instance, your **mouth** is very important part for several reasons: your smile is very important in being sexually attractive to your husband, your mouth is the part you use for kissing, and your mouth is the part you use to perform fellatio. Your **tongue** is important in kissing, fellatio, and other erotic behavior such as thrusting your tongue in and out of your husband's ear. Surprise, your **hands** are a very important part of your body for sexual activity; they provide stimulation to both you and your husband. And, your **anus** can be a major source of sexual pleasure to you when stimulated by narrow things such as fingers and some types of toys, and can provide pleasure to your husband as an alternative to vaginal intercourse.

The **G-spot** is an erogenous area on the front wall of the vagina, and some women are more sensitive than others when pressure is applied there. Recent research indicates that the pleasure derived from G-spot manipulation may be due to that pressure being felt by the small **para-urethral gland**, which surrounds the urethra and is the source of female ejaculation fluid. Interestingly, some women who get no significant pleasure from pressure on the G-spot do get pleasure from downward pressure on their **mons pubis**, and that may be another, more indirect way of applying pressure to the para-urethral gland.

There are other erotic areas of the female body, which are mentioned in the section on Erogenous Zones a little later, but these are some of the most important ones.

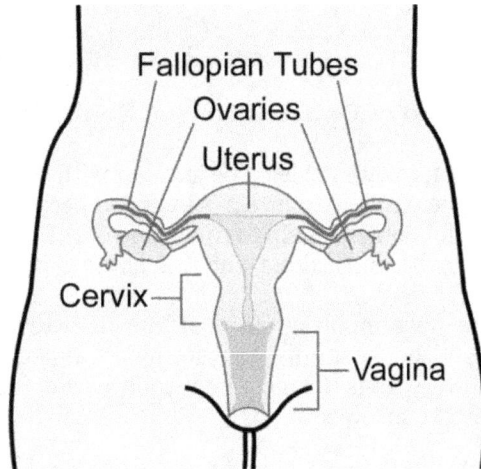

Figure 3. Front-Sectional View of Female Reproductive Organs

Just as it's important for you to be familiar with your sexual organs, you also need to be familiar with a woman's reproductive cycle, because it can affect your ability to get aroused and can be an issue regarding birth control, which is covered in the section on pregnancy.

The Female Reproductive Cycle

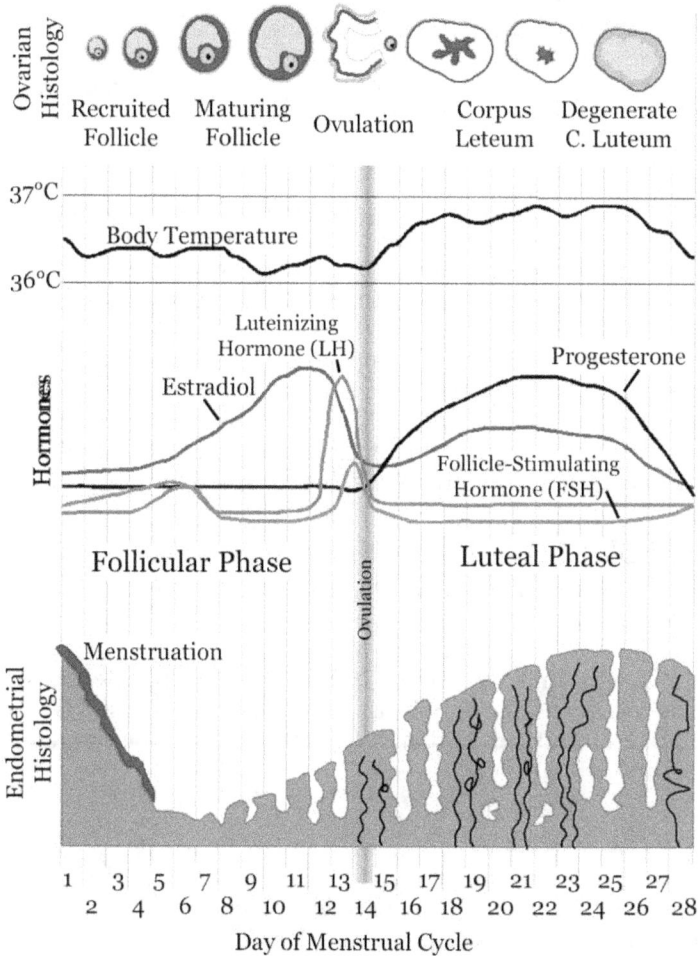

Figure 4. Reproductive/Menstrual Cycle[5]
*Average values for days. Durations and values may differ
between different females or different cycles.*

A woman's reproductive period begins toward the end of
puberty and ends with menopause. In between, the menstrual
cycle controls when you can become pregnant. The typical
idealized menstrual cycle is 28 days long, but it usually varies
from cycle to cycle, and it can vary by a few days to more than
20.

---

[5] You can find a larger, color version of this image at Wikipedia
under the topic of "Menstrual cycle".

Menstrual Phase, Days 1–4

If you haven't become pregnant during the past menstrual cycle, a new cycle begins in which your uterus sheds it's lining. When it begins, small amounts of blood are eliminated through your vagina. The amount of blood increases, reaches a maximum, then diminishes and quits.

If you have intercourse during days of heavy bleeding, the amount of blood coming out is usually enough to require extra care. This particular problem can be dealt with simply by having sex in the shower or lying down with a maxi pad under you.

Many women prefer not to have sexual intercourse during menstruation, and Islam bans it, but there is no known medical reason to avoid it. One advantage to having intercourse during menstruation is that it's extremely unlikely that you'll get pregnant, even if no birth control is used.

Follicular / Proliferative Phase, Days 5–13

Each ovarian follicle contains a single ovum (egg), and in this phase, one or more follicles mature.

Many women experience heightened sexual desire in this phase, especially in the several days immediately before ovulation, perhaps due to increases in the estradiol, LH, or FSH hormones.

Ovulation, Day 14

Ovulation is when an ovarian follicle releases an ovum into your fallopian tubes. This is not considered a phase, but an event dividing the Follicular and Luteal phases.

Luteal / Secretory Phase, Days 15–26

During this phase, the ovarian follicle that released an ovum is transformed into a corpus luteum which secretes hormones.

Ischemic Phase, Days 27–28

Often considered part of the luteal phase, this 1 or 2 day period is characterized by estradiol and progesterone diminishing rapidly to their lowest points and the constriction of the spiral arteries of the endometrium. The ischemia results in shrinkage and degeneration of the endometrium.

Fertile Period

Your fertile period is the time with the highest likelihood of becoming pregnant.

To become pregnant, you must have a viable sperm inside your uterus at the same time as a viable ovum. Since an ovum is usually viable for about 2 days after ovulation, and sperm are typically viable inside a woman from 1-5 days (with a maximum of about 8 days), your fertile period is from several days to a week before ovulation to about 2 days after.

Note that it can be difficult to predict exactly when you will ovulate, especially if your periods are very irregular. This can impact your plans if you're trying to get pregnant, or if you're trying to use the timing method of birth control.

Female Erogenous Zones

An erogenous zone is a sensitive area of the human body that results in a sexual response when stimulated.

Any part of your body and every part of your body can create sensual feelings, but some are more commonly sensitive than others. Some are highly sensitive all the time, while some are sensitive only when you are highly aroused. Sensitivity varies from woman to woman, and it varies over time for the same woman.

Stimulating an erogenous zone requires movement of some kind, and are commonly manual stroking with moderate or heavy pressure, and feather-light touches.

The clitoris has the most dense nerve supply of any part of the skin and provides the most erogenous zone on the female body. Here are all of the most common erogenous zones in women, grouped by Grandma Synthia from most sensitive to least:

1. Clitoris.
2. Anus, breasts, clitoral hood, lips, nipples.
3. Areola, inner thighs, labia, perineum.
4. A-spot, ears, G-spot, neck, U-spot.
5. Fingers, souls of the feet, toes, tongue.

Female Sexual Response Cycle

The four-phases of physiological responses to sexual stimulation are the excitement phase, plateau phase, orgasmic phase, and resolution phase.

Excitement Phase

This phase is characterized by sexual arousal, and includes both physical and mental aspects.

A woman may experience arousal at any time, but many women have increased sexual desire in the several days immediately before ovulation.

When something in a woman's physical environment or something in her thoughts begins to cause a sexual reaction, her body and mind respond in specific ways.

The primary physical reactions are that blood flow increases in the vaginal walls, the vagina begins to secret a lubricating fluid, the clitoris and labia begin to swell, nipples become erect, and erogenous zones become more sensitive to touch. In addition, the heart rate, blood pressure, and breathing rate increase, the skin may flush, breasts may increase slightly in size, the cervix and uterus elevate, the depth of the vagina slightly increases as the cervix elevates, and the labia may change in shape and color.

The immediate primary mental reaction is increased awareness of the sexual stimulation and a decision (consciously or subconsciously) to pursue or evade the stimulation. If the decision is to pursue the stimulation, then thoughts begin to focus on how to continue and increase the stimulation. If the initial stimulation is from sexual thoughts, then increasing the stimulation may involve the addition of physical stimulation. If the initial stimulation is physical, then increasing the stimulation may involve physical stimulation to more sensitive erogenous areas or the addition of sexual thoughts. Regardless of the initial type of stimulation, consideration may be given to improving the sexual suitability of the environment, such as seeking privacy.

Activities associated with the excitement phase can include flirting, reading romantic or sexually suggestive or explicit literature, imagining erotic scenarios (initial fantasizing), viewing erotic images, listening to erotic sounds, light kissing, light touching of non-genital areas, or breast-feeding.

The excitement phase typically lasts a few minutes, but may last anywhere from seconds to days, and eventually terminates or escalates to the plateau phase.

Plateau Phase

Continued sexual activity becomes more intimate and more active physically, and more imaginative mentally.

Physical changes include reaching a maximum sensitivity to touch, increased touching and movement, increased pleasure from touching and movement, increases in muscle tension, increases in circulation and heart rate, and the production of endorphins in the brain. In addition, the areola and labia further increase in size, the clitoris withdraws slightly, the vagina continues to produce lubrication, the vagina swells, and the pubococcygeus muscle tightens, reducing the diameter of the opening of the vagina. Women may also begin to moan or vocalize involuntarily.

Mental changes may include increased awareness of physical pleasure, decrease in awareness of chronic pain (if any), a diminishing or loss of awareness of physical surroundings, a diminishing or loss of higher reasoning skills, or conscious or subconscious decisions to pursue thoughts or physical changes to increase physical pleasure, delay orgasm, or initiate orgasm.

Activities associated with the plateau phase include undressing, touching or massaging genitals or other intimate erotic areas (heavy petting), passionate kissing, French kissing, increase in the explicitness of sexual fantasy, rapid changes in sexual fantasies, explicit sex talk, oral sex, or sexual intercourse of any kind.

Orgasmic Phase

Orgasm is the conclusion of the plateau phase and is characterized by rapid contractions of the uterus, vagina, and the lower pelvic muscles surrounding the anus and the vagina. Orgasms often include involuntary moaning, muscular spasms in other areas of the body, and a generally euphoric sensation. Orgasms may also play a role in fertilization, as it is theorized that the muscular spasms may aid in the locomotion of spermatozoa up the vaginal walls into the uterus.

Some women experience a female ejaculation of a liquid originating from the paraurethral gland, which has tubes that empty into the urethra. Although women can be incontinent (leaking urine) when they have an orgasm, female ejaculate fluid includes only trace amounts of urine, and unlike urine, it includes prostate-specific antigens (PSA).

Many women have difficulty experiencing orgasms, and psychological attitude and DNA may both be factors. Research into helping such women achieve orgasms is a growing field, with some signs of promise for medications for average women and spinal cord stimulation for more extreme cases.

For most women, **the most rapid way to reach an orgasm is through direct, continuous stimulation of the clitoris**, especially by the husband's tongue. How long it takes to reach an orgasm may depend on how long it's been since the last one, and the quality and duration of the excitement phase.

In tantric sex, an ancient Indian spiritual tradition (not associated with Tantric Buddhism), orgasms are avoided or postponed as long as possible in order to increase the enjoyment of the plateau phase.

> **The clitoris has the most dense nerve supply of any part of the skin and provides the most erogenous zone on the female body.**

Resolution Phase

The resolution phase occurs after orgasm and allows the muscles to relax, blood pressure to drop and the body to slow down from its excited state.

Most women experience a recovery period after orgasm during which it is physiologically impossible to have additional orgasms, and during which continued stimulation may be unpleasant or mildly painful. Recovery periods can vary greatly from person to person and over time for the same person, but are generally in the range of half an hour to several hours.

With practice, some women have been able to learn to control their resolution so that they return immediately to the plateau stage and are capable of achieving another orgasm quickly. This is referred as being multi-orgasmic.

The Male World

Male Anatomy

Now comes your husband's plumbing. Once you're married, his assets are your assets, and you should get to know them as well as he does, or better!

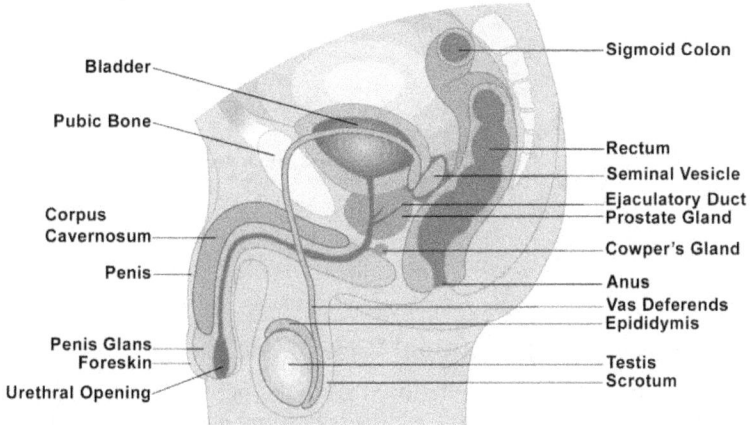

Figure 5. Cross-Sectional View of Male Pelvic Organs

Figure 5 shows a man's pelvic area. His external genitals consist of his penis and scrotum.

You can learn to feel your husband's scrotum for abnormal lumps and help him practice regular health checkups for testicular cancer that way. If he's had a vasectomy, there will two pea-sized lumps. Be gentle, because squeezing his testicles too hard is very painful.

Another health check you can do for your husband, if you're willing, is to check his prostate gland for hardness or lumps. This requires inserting a well-lubricated index finger into his rectum and pressing along the front wall. The prostate is normally walnut sized and has a medium firmness. One mild caution here is that the prostate gland is an erogenous zone, so after performing this check, he might want you to perform something else! Wash your hands, of course, unless you use medical gloves, which you can buy inexpensive at any pharmacy.

Grandma Anne recommends performing both of these checks at
the same time, on the first day of each month. How will you
know if something's abnormal? Well, you start doing it, and by
doing it many times while it's normal, you'll learn what normal
feels like. Once you know what normal feels like, you'll be able
to tell if any lumps appear in the testicles or prostate, or hard
spots in the prostate. You can check each other's breasts for
lumps, also. Remember that men can also get breast cancer.

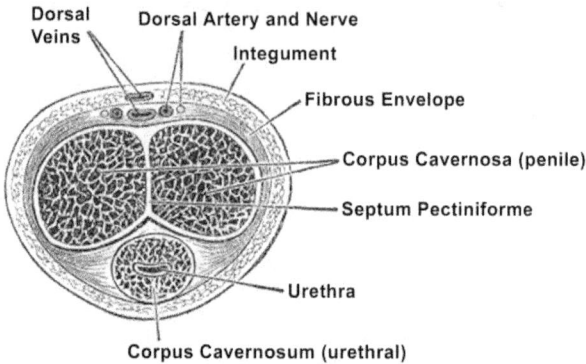

Figure 6. Cross-Sectional View of Penis

Figure 6 shows a cross sectional view of a penis, including the
urethra. Though a woman's clitoris is somewhat analogous to a
man's penis, the urethra does not go through a woman's clitoris,
but it goes through the entire length of a man's penis. The
urethra is what urine comes out of, so that's why men can pee
standing up and aim when they pee.

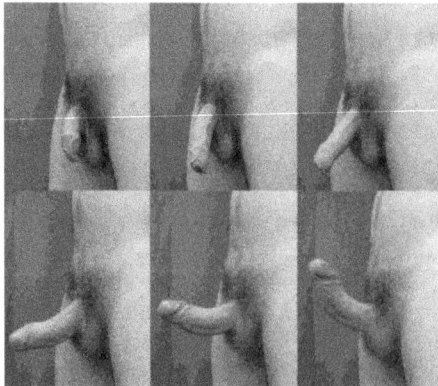

Figure 7. Process of Erection, Uncircumcised Penis

So you can know what to expect on your honeymoon, figure 7
shows the foreskin withdrawing from the head of a penis as it
becomes erect.

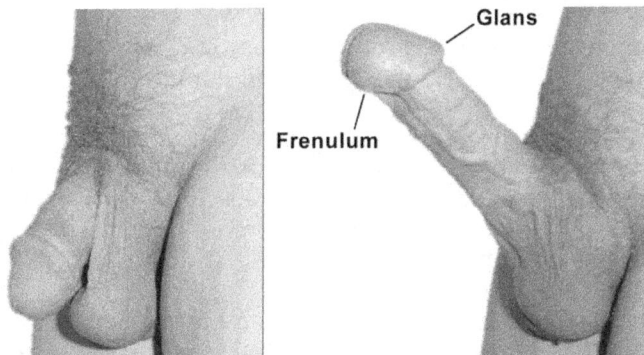

Figure 8. Circumcised Penis, Flaccid and Erect

Since figure 7 shows an uncircumcised penis becoming erect, figure 8 shows the before and after of a circumcised penis. Circumcision is the surgical removal of the foreskin, so the head of a circumcised penis is never covered by that extra skin. Comparing figures 7 and 8, you can see that some penises curve, and some are straight. Figure 8 also clearly distinguishes between the glans and the frenulum, which are the most sensitive parts of the penis.

Semen

Semen is a fluid containing sperm and seminal plasma, and is produced by secretions of the seminal vesicle, prostate, and Cowper's (bulbourethral) glands. It is excreted through the penis in the process of ejaculation and typically is 1 or 2 tablespoons (10-20 milliliters) in volume. Lower volumes may occur after very frequent ejaculation and higher volumes are seen after prolonged abstinence.

One ejaculation may have over 1,000,000,000 (1 billion) sperm. In healthy, fertile men, it is normal for about 25% of sperm to be dead when ejaculated.

Sperm take over 70 days to develop, are produced solely in the testicles, and pass through the epididymis before they can be ejaculated. They resemble tadpoles with very long tales.

Sperm count in the average male is anywhere between 20 million and 150 million sperm per milliliter, and if the sperm count is below 20 million per milliliter, infertility is likely.

Male Erogenous Zones

An erogenous zone is a sensitive area of the human body that results in a sexual response when stimulated.

Any part of a man's body can create sensual feelings, but some are more commonly sensitive than others. Some are highly sensitive all the time, while some are sensitive only when he is highly aroused, and this sensitivity varies from man to man, and it varies over time for the same man.

Stimulating an erogenous zone requires movement of some kind, and are commonly manual stroking with moderate or heavy pressure, and feather-light touches.

The head of the penis has the most dense nerve supply of any part of the skin and provides the most erogenous zone on the male body. Here are the most common erogenous zones in men, based on Grandma Synthia's assessment, and grouped from most sensitive to least:

1. Frenulum, Penis glans.
2. Anus, ears, lips, P-spot.
3. Perineum, tongue.
4. Necks.

As indicated by this list compared to the erogenous zones listed for women, the average man is sexually sensitized to less of his body than the average woman. In addition, a woman's clitoris has a higher density of nerves than the head of a man's penis.

Male Sexual Response Cycle

The four phases of physiological responses to sexual stimulation are the excitement phase, plateau phase, orgasmic phase, and resolution phase.

Excitement/Arousal Phase

This phase is characterized by sexual arousal, and includes both physical and mental aspects.

A man may experience arousal at any time, and men generally get aroused more often and more easily than women. Most sexually suggestive advertising is intended to arouse men, and the most sensitive part of their penis is subjected to friction from their clothes whenever their legs move.

Your husband may not tell you when he needs sex, or how much he needs it. Until you learn his sexual needs well, or he tells you he doesn't need a sexual release, assume he does if it's been more than 24 hours.

When something in a man's physical environment or something in his thoughts begins to cause a sexual reaction, his body and mind respond in specific ways.

The primary physical reactions are increased blood flow to the corpus cavernosa, which initiates a full or partial erection of the penis, often after only a few seconds of erotic stimulation. During an erection, the urinary bladder closes and prevents urine from mixing with semen. The erection may be partially lost and regained repeatedly during an extended excitement phase. In addition to an erection, the heart rate, blood pressure, and breathing rate increase, the skin may flush, pre-ejaculatory fluid begins to leak from the penis, the testicles swell and are drawn upward, and the scrotum can tense and thicken. In about 60% of men, an erection of the nipples will occur.

As with women, the immediate primary mental reaction is increased awareness of the sexual stimulation and a decision (consciously or subconsciously) to pursue or evade the stimulation. If the decision is to pursue the stimulation, then thoughts begin to focus on how to continue and increase the stimulation. If the initial stimulation is from sexual thoughts, then increasing the stimulation may involve the addition of physical stimulation. If the initial stimulation is physical, then increasing the stimulation may involve physical stimulation to more sensitive erogenous areas or the addition of sexual thoughts. Regardless of the initial type of stimulation, consideration may be given to improving the sexual suitability of the environment, such as seeking privacy.

Activities associated with the excitement phase can include flirting, reading romantic or sexually suggestive or explicit literature, imagining erotic scenarios (initial fantasizing), viewing erotic images, listening to erotic sounds, light kissing, or light touching of non-genital areas.

The excitement phase typically lasts a few minutes, but may last anywhere from seconds to hours, and eventually terminates or escalates to the plateau phase.

Plateau Phase

Continued sexual activity becomes more intimate and more active physically, and more imaginative mentally.

Physical changes include reaching a maximum sensitivity to touch, increased touching and movement, increased pleasure from touching and movement, increases in muscle tension, increases in circulation and heart rate, and the production of endorphins in the brain. In addition, the release of pre-ejaculatory fluid increases, and muscles at the base of the penis may begin rhythmic contractions. Men may also begin to moan or vocalize involuntarily.

Mental changes may include increased awareness of physical pleasure, decrease in awareness of chronic pain (if any), a diminishing or loss of awareness of physical surroundings, a diminishing or loss of higher reasoning skills, or conscious or subconscious decisions to pursue thoughts or physical changes to increase physical pleasure (friction on the head of the penis), delay orgasm, or initiate orgasm.

Activities associated with the plateau phase include undressing, touching or massaging genitals or other intimate erotic areas (heavy petting), passionate kissing, French kissing, increase in the explicitness of sexual fantasy, rapid changes in sexual fantasies, explicit sex talk, oral sex, or sexual intercourse of any kind.

Orgasmic Phase

Orgasm is the conclusion of the plateau phase and is characterized by ejaculation of semen in several spurts. Each spurt is associated with a wave of sexual pleasure, especially in the head of the penis. The first and second convulsions are usually the most intense in sensation, and produce the greatest quantity of semen. Thereafter, each contraction is associated with a diminishing volume of semen and a milder wave of pleasure. In addition, a male orgasm is usually accompanied by contractions in the pelvic muscles surrounding both the anus and the penis. Orgasms often include involuntary moaning, muscular spasms in other areas of the body, and a generally euphoric sensation.

For most men, the most rapid way to reach an orgasm is through direct, lubricated stimulation of the head of the penis (the glans and frenulum) accompanied by real, simulated, or imagined orgasm by a woman. How long it takes to reach an orgasm may depend on how long it has been since the last one, and on the quality and duration of the excitement and plateau phases.

In tantric sex, an ancient Indian spiritual tradition (not associated with Tantric Buddhism), orgasms are avoided or postponed as long as possible in order to increase the enjoyment of the plateau phase.

Resolution Phase

The resolution phase occurs after orgasm and allows the muscles to relax, blood pressure to drop and the body to slow down from its excited state.

Most men experience a recovery period after orgasm during which it is physiologically impossible to have additional orgasms, and during which continued stimulation may be unpleasant or mildly painful. Recovery periods can vary greatly from person to person and over time for the same person, but are generally much shorter than for women, and can range from a few minutes to an hour.

> **There are two spots on the head of the penis that are especially sensitive:**
> **The Frenulum and the Glans.**

Types Of Sex

Teasing / Flirting

Some folks consider flirting as innocent, some don't. If you're married and someone's flirting with your spouse, you're *not* likely to see it as an innocent activity. If your spouse is flirting with someone else, you're likely to get angry.

Grandma Synthia believes that it should be obvious: flirting is intended to create sexual arousal, and is a prelude to physical interaction. If you aren't intending to have sex, it's dangerous, because you might end up having sex and expressing bewilderment as to how it could have happened, just like millions of people before you.

So, don't flirt with anyone other than your spouse. But with your spouse, flirt all the time!

Foreplay / Petting

Foreplay, also known as petting, is physical touching that causes sexual arousal.

Yes, it's true... many, many, many people have believed that there's nothing wrong with "light" petting between single people, such as kissing, as long as it goes no further. And they believe that right up until the time they get pregnant and wonder how that happened. And many people continue to think there's nothing wrong with kissing and caressing even after they've ended up having sex many times when they didn't intend to.

Grandma Synthia says that the problem isn't with a kiss itself, it's that a kiss will be so pleasant it will create a very strong desire for something more intimate, such as a caress of the breast. And that will be so pleasant it will create a very strong desire for something even more intimate, and on and on.

If you're a Christian, and you seriously want to avoid having sex before marriage, then *don't touch*! Even simple, innocent little hand-holding can start you on a sexual meltdown (see page 14).

Once you get married, though, yahoo! Pet each other all the time! Foreplay leading to sex can last seconds or days, and the anticipation is wonderful.

> **Grandma Caroline:** *My husband and I enjoy foreplay almost as much as we enjoy sex itself. For us, foreplay for the next episode of sex starts right after one episode of sex ends. If we've not having it, we're planning it.*

You can have sex spontaneously, but you can also schedule specific days and times for sex. Some Grandmas like to occasionally set a date and time and then have a countdown, with the intervening kisses, hugs, and intimate caresses becoming more and more frequent, and with a whispered count of how many hours or minutes remain. There is one problem with this technique though: We often don't last until the scheduled time before we end up well beyond the foreplay phase!

Manual Sex

No, we don't mean masturbation, although many people do use the term manual sex to refer to masturbation. We refer to masturbation as... *masturbation*, and a subsequent chapter is devoted to that topic.

We mean "manual" as in "hands". As in a wife using her hands to stroke up and down her husband's penis, or a husband using his fingers to stroke his wife's clitoris or insert them into her vagina, all intended to bring the spouse to an orgasm or at least get them closer to it.

Inserting a well-lubricated finger into the anus can also be very stimulating, especially for the man if his wife touches the P-Spot. Just remember to wear medical gloves or thoroughly wash your hands before putting them anywhere else.

Oral Sex

Oral sex means the wife putting her husband's penis in her mouth (fellatio) or licking his penis or testicles, or the husband putting his mouth on his wife's genitals, especially his tongue to her clitoris (cunnilingus).

BASIC SEX

If you want your husband to get an erection as quickly as possible, use your mouth on his penis. If his penis has deflated because he's had an orgasm recently, you can often easily get him re-inflated with fellatio. Fellatio is also known by many slang terms, the most common of which is probably "blow-job". You don't actually blow, however, you lick and suck.

If you wake up and want to have sex, see if your husband's in a position that allows you to get your mouth on his penis. No matter how tired he is, he's not likely to complain about being woken up this way!

If you want to have an orgasm as quickly as possible, the easiest way for most women is for their husbands to lick their clitoris, either in a very steady rhythm, or at a very slowly increasing pace. This is cunnilingus, which is also known by many slang terms, including "blow-job" and "muff-diving", but the most common is probably "eating pussy". You can ask your husband to do this any way you want to, but nothing is more direct or to-the-point than "please eat me." That kind of assertive request is a huge turn-on for many men.

Did you know that oral sex is in the Bible? It sure is, in the Bible's sex book, the Song of Songs (also known as the Song of Solomon), chapter 7, verse 2. It's camouflaged, though, because all the people who translated the Bible into English translated the word for vagina as "navel" or "waist", and the word for labia usually as "waist" or "belly". Well, if all the translators translated it those ways, how do we know different? If they all agree, that's pretty reliable isn't it? No, because almost all published Bible commentators agree that vagina and labia are what the original language in Hebrew means. We'll come back to this issue after you read the passage:

Song of Songs, 7:1-6
How beautiful are your sandaled feet, O prince's daughter! Your graceful legs are like jewels, the work of a craftsman's hands. Your navel is a rounded goblet that never lacks blended wine. Your waist is a mound of wheat encircled by lilies. Your breasts are like two fawns, twins of a gazelle. Your neck is like an ivory tower. Your eyes are the pools of Heshbon by the gate of Bath Rabbim. Your nose is like the tower of Lebanon looking toward Damascus. Your head crowns you like Mount Carmel. Your hair is like royal tapestry; the king is held captive by its tresses. How beautiful you are and how pleasing, O love, with your delights!

Now if the translators were right, and the commentators are wrong, how does the Lover in this passage get mixed wine from a navel?? As Marvin H. Pope, author of *Song of Songs : Anchor Bible Commentary*, points out, "navels are not notable for their capacity to store or dispense moisture".

Besides, the Lover is describing the most notable parts of a woman in a very erotic way. Do you seriously think he's going to mention belly button and waist and not mention or even allude to her genitals?! Grandma Synthia is convinced the true list of the physical attributes the Lover recites are: feet, thighs, vagina, labia, breasts, neck, eyes, nose, head, hair. Oh, yeah!

The original writing was in the Hebrew language, and the word translated as "navel" is *shor*. Bible commentator Cheryl Exum notes that "Some suggest that *shor* is metonymy for vulva because of its proximity to it and because it resembles an aperture (Krinetzki, Longman; on the interchangeability of navel and vulva in ancient Near Eastern iconography, see Keel, figs. 127, 104-7)."[6]

Grandma Dora has studied this extensively, and suggests the most accurate translation of the vagina sentence is:

Your vagina is perfectly formed like a goblet filled with mixed wine.

What's all this got to do with oral sex? Well, Grandma Dora likes to point out that **this clearly implies that the Lover knows what his Beloved's vagina *tastes* like.** You can recognize wine by seeing it or smelling it, but you can't recognize mixed wine without *tasting* it.

Vaginal Intercourse

Vaginal intercourse means a penis inside a vagina. The husband can thrust in and out, or the wife can "ride" up and down or back and forth, depending on their positions.

This is the most intuitive form of intercourse, especially combined with the missionary position, and therefore doesn't need a lot of explanation here. When an inexperienced man and woman start out petting and end up having sex without

[6] Exum, J. Cheryl (2005). *Song of Songs: A Commentary*. Louisville, Kentucky: Westminster John Knox Press

planning for it, this is how they're most like to end up doing it. Couples also tend to keep doing it this way until they get used to it and start experimenting with other positions and other forms of intercourse.

Anal Intercourse

Anal intercourse takes getting used to, and some women just can't seem to get used to it *mentally*.

Based on Grandma Yvette's experience as a professional prostitute, before she became a Christian, all men like anal sex at least occasionally, some men prefer it over vaginal intercourse, and some men prefer to begin intercourse in the vagina but switch to the anus to have their orgasm.

Based on Yvette's conversations with many colleagues, most women feared it before they ever tried it, and most of the women who hadn't been taught how to deal with it hated it after they tried it because the men used no lubrication, too little lubrication, or jammed it in without getting the sphincter muscle relaxed first. Because men pay prostitutes for sexual satisfaction, and because so many men want anal sex, most prostitutes eventually learn to at least tolerate it. According to Yvette, some married men come to prostitutes primarily because their wives wouldn't have anal sex with them.

Grandma Yvette also points out that some women come to enjoy anal sex, including herself. In fact, there is a technique she enjoys where her husband wears a strap-on dildo so he can penetrate both her vagina and anus at the same time. There are several options for this, such as when sometimes she'll be face down and her husband will wear a slender dildo above his penis, so that he penetrates her vagina and the dildo penetrates her anus. At other times, she lays face up, and her husband penetrates her anus with his penis and a thicker dildo penetrates her vagina.

If you decide to try anal intercourse, you need to use a *lot* of lubricant and get the anal sphincter muscle warmed up before penal penetration.

The first few times you have anal sex, the husband should first insert a well lubricated finger into your anus and wait, or move slowly back and forth, perhaps for several minutes, until he feels your anal sphincter muscle relax. This is anal *stimulation*, as opposed to intercourse. Many people enjoy this as part of their love-making even if they don't have anal intercourse. After it relaxes, he can withdraw his finger and *slowly* insert his well lubricated penis. After awhile, you'll learn how to relax that muscle some, and he won't need to use his finger as long as he still uses plenty of lubricant. Water or oil-based lubricants can work, but silicone-based lubricant will last longer, which will help since the rectum doesn't provide much natural moisture.

And, anal sex is not just for men! You can strap on a dildo and "peg" your husband's anus, enhancing your ability to pretend you're a man, and enhancing his ability to pretend he's a woman, which is known as gender-reversal role-playing. In addition, penetrating your husband's anus with a finger, dildo, or vibrating butt-plug is the best way to stimulate his P-Spot (prostate gland), which can significantly increase his pleasure.

Dispelling Anal Sex Myths

- Anal sex will not permanently stretch your anus so that it won't close properly anymore. It will take five minutes or more after anal sex before it fully returns to normal closure, but it will.
- Allowing your husband to penetrate your anus does *not* mean he's homosexual, and it won't turn him into one.
- If you're healthy, your rectum normally doesn't have much fecal matter until a few minutes before you need to have a bowel movement, so that doesn't interfere.

Warning: Never go from anus to vagina or from anus to mouth with *anything* without thoroughly washing it first, and *never* practice "rimming", which is stimulation of the anus with your tongue. The anus has a lot of bacteria that can cause serious infections when it gets in other places.

Note: Islamic law universally condemns anal sex, and there are many "Prophetic traditions" which state that. However, all these traditions appear to be traced back to a single sentence in the Quran: "Your wives are as a tilth unto you; so approach your tilth when and how you will" (2:223) "Tilth" means a place to cultivate, or a place to put your seed. That clearly asserts that it is permissible for a man to have vaginal sex, but it does not assert anything at all about having sex with your wife in a manner not intended to get her pregnant. It doesn't say that anal sex is permissible or impermissible, because it doesn't say anything about it at all. The near-universal *interpretation* that this passage prohibits anal sex is clearly wrong.

Other Forms Of Sex

Other forms of stimulating a man's penis to the point of orgasm include:

- **Armpit Intercourse**, sliding a penis in and out of a woman's armpit.
- **Cameltoe Stroking**, a woman on top, sliding her labia up and down a penis, pressing the penis against the man's abdomen.
- **Crotch Intercourse**, sliding a penis between a woman's thighs and touching the labia.
- **Mammary Intercourse**, sliding a penis between a woman's breasts.
- **Waist Stroking**, when a man pins his penis between his and his wife's waists as he slides back and forth.

Other forms of stimulating a woman to the point of orgasm include:

- **Rhino Stroking**, a man in a 69 position using his nose to caress the woman's labia and the entrance to her vagina while performing cunnilingus. The first inch or so of the vaginal canal has a greater concentration of nerve endings than the deeper parts.
- **Hump-Rub**, the woman manually stroking her clitoris, or near it, while her husband performs vaginal intercourse. This is very erotic to most men, and often gets them to an orgasm faster.
- **Pounding**, using a position that allows the penis to penetrate the vagina so that the tip touches or hits the back end of the vagina (the A-Spot). This is not possible for a couple where the penis doesn't reach to the back of the vagina.

Grandma Brenda: Sometimes my husband has to work at it [vaginal intercourse] a long time before he can climax, and it's common for us to change positions several times. One night in our first year of marriage, we changed positions, and when he started getting close to a climax, he started thrusting much harder, and it really hurt! I didn't say anything, because I wanted him to be able to finish, and I didn't want to disappoint him, but it hurt so much I couldn't keep from crying. I was quiet, though, and he was so caught up in what he was doing that he didn't notice. He finally finished and collapsed on top of me, and I was able to wipe my tears away before he noticed. I

*had trouble getting to sleep that night, and I
wondered if that would ever happen again, and if so,
whether or not I'd be able to do my duty long enough
for him to finish. I was still troubled the next morning,
and I was <u>sore</u>. I had never been anywhere near that
sore, and it hurt with every step I took.*

*Well, it took several days before the soreness wore off,
and it was just after that when it happened again.
This time, he only did it for about a minute before he
finished, so it didn't last so long.*

*The next day, I was sore again, but it wasn't as bad.
Now this may seem silly, but I felt like a heroine. I had
done battle in the bedroom to satisfy my husband,
and I had succeeded, even though it cost a little pain. I
actually strutted around the house, feeling the
soreness with every step, and I was enjoying it!
Nevertheless, I anxiously awaited the next time it
might happen, not knowing how it would turn out.*

*Well, it happened again very soon, and as soon as he
made one powerful thrust that hit me hard, I
involuntarily cried out with an "ow" or something like
that, and my husband immediately stopped.*

*I thought in that first moment that I had really failed in
my sexual duties, and many bad thoughts flashed
through my mind about how my husband would be
disappointed with me for the rest of our lives.*

*Well, my loving husband realized what had caused
my cry, and he apologized, and we had a long talk,
mostly about him wanting me to tell him if he ever did
anything that hurt me.*

*It was hard for me, but I learned how to tell him when
I had a problem, and together we learned how to
adjust to each other, including learning how he could
thrust into me really hard without hitting the back of
my vagina too hard.*

*Well, that was wonderful, but it wasn't quite the end
of that story. I learned in some positions how to
adjust my body so I could control whether or not he
hit the back of my vagina, and with how much force.
And... I came to really, really, like it when it was just
right. And every time I have it just right, I go
strutting around the house the next day, savoring
every footstep!*

None of us other Grandmas were familiar with "pounding" as a
sexual technique until Grandma Elizabeth discovered it while
researching. We had all experienced an occasional thrust that

went too deep, too hard, but it was always painful, not something to lead to orgasm. After Elizabeth found reports that some women claimed they were able to come to orgasm based on pounding, we discussed it, but initially decided not to include it in this book, because we didn't trust the information.

Nothing else was said about it after that, until one day when Grandma Brenda raised the subject again and shyly admitted how she had come to enjoy it on a regular basis, even though it didn't get her to orgasm. The fact that it was Grandma Brenda intrigued us, as she was the least inclined among us to experiment, and seemed to have an abnormally low libido. How could she have stumbled onto something that the rest of us had missed, and never even heard of?

Well, we decided to give it further consideration, which meant a bunch of other Grandmas needed to experiment with it first-hand. Here are our very non-scientific conclusions:

Pounding can be difficult to get used to, as it can be quite painful with too much force, or if done for too long. However, it is possible to get used to it, and to become proficient at controlling the force applied, primarily by fine-tuning the position of your hips. There are two possible benefits. First, it can create a mild soreness that is definitely erotic, such as Grandma Brenda related. Secondly, it is definitely possible for it to lead to an orgasm. For those of us who were able to get to an orgasm this way, we rated it a 10-out-of-10.

Lubricants and oils can make sex more fun, but not if they're too cold!

When you start getting in the mood, fill the sink in your bathroom with hot water and put your bottles or tubes of lube and oil in the water. When they go on warm, your libido will stay hot!

Sex Positions

Which positions are good for sex? Any position that gets the penis into the vagina will do. Or the mouth to whatever part you're trying to get it to. Use your imagination.

Why do people try different positions? Because different positions create slightly different sensations for the husband or wife. Curiosity spurs us to try them all, and we usually find a few favorites that we like to stick with for a long time, and then from time to time we replace an old favorite with a new favorite.

There are an almost endless combination of options, including lying down, kneeling, standing up, side-by-side, front-to-back, face-up, and face-down. Many positions put the man in control, many put the woman in control, and many others allow either spouse to be in control or to share control. By "in control" we're referring to the person controlling the depth of the thrusts during intercourse.

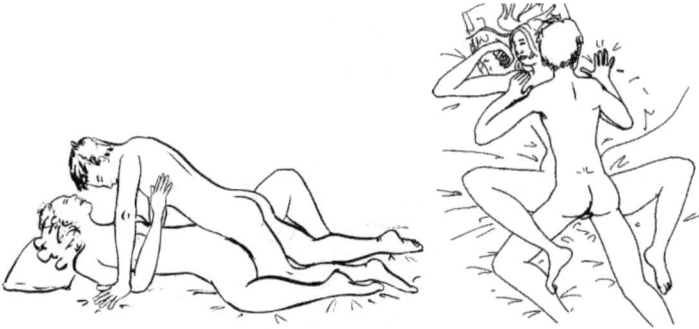

Figure 9. Missionary positions

Missionary positions are the most common for beginners, with the woman lying face-up and the man lying on top.

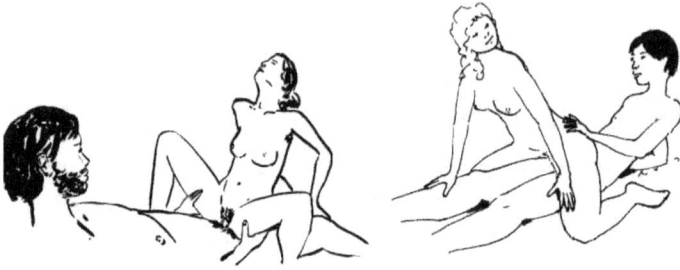

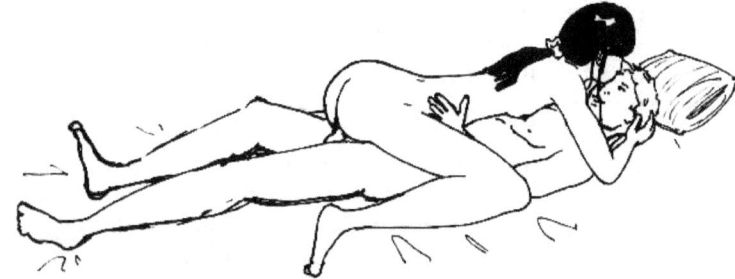

Figure 10. Amazon positions

Amazon positions involve the wife on top, facing her husband, and reverse-Amazon has her on top facing away from her husband.

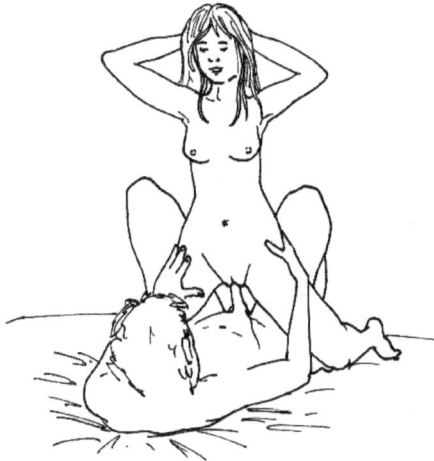

Figure 11. Cowgirl position

The Cowgirl position is an Amazon-position, but with the wife moving her pelvis as if she's riding a horse.

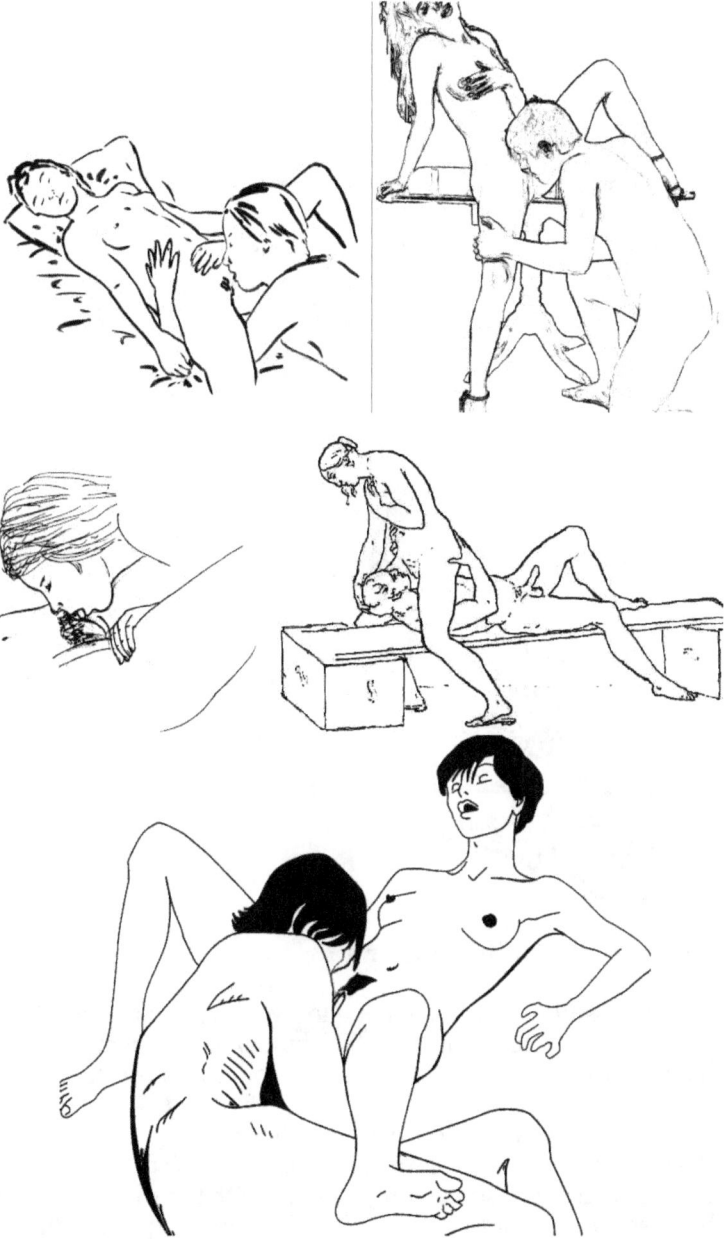

Figure 12. Cunnilingus positions

Cunnilingus positions are those that allow your husband to lick your clitoris with his tongue, or to insert his tongue into your vagina.

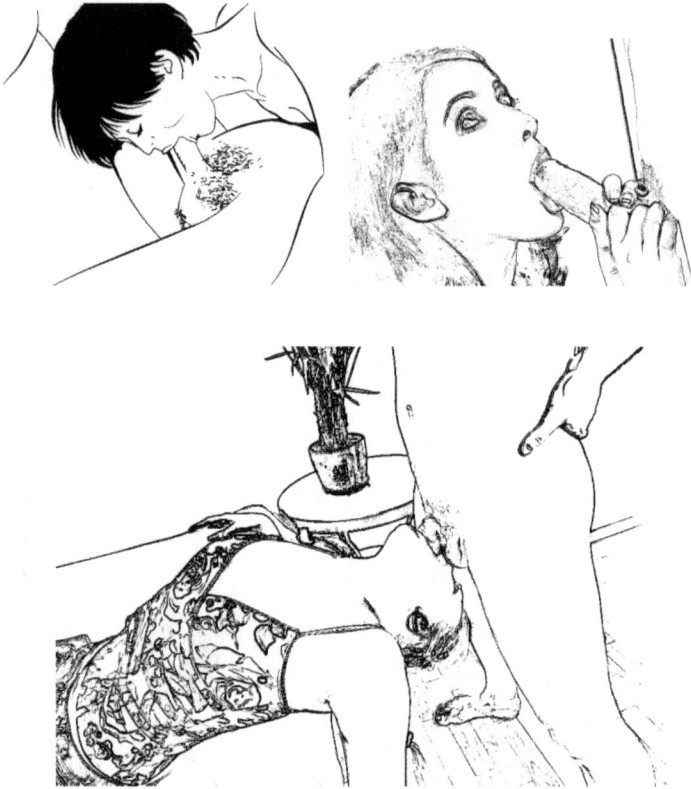

Figure 13. Fellatio positions

Fellatio positions are those that allow you to put your mouth on your husband's penis, or that allow him to put his penis in your mouth. The difference is which one of you is in control.

Deep-throating is fellatio where your husband's penis goes past the back of your mouth, into the top part of your throat. This takes practice, and should only be done with the wife in control, because you may not be able to breathe when his penis is fully inserted. Most women find this to be the most difficult sex tip to master, and some never do. Husbands love it, of course, and women who are able to master this like it because it gets such a big reaction from their husband, and it allows them to swallow an ejaculation without tasting it (it's usually very salty).

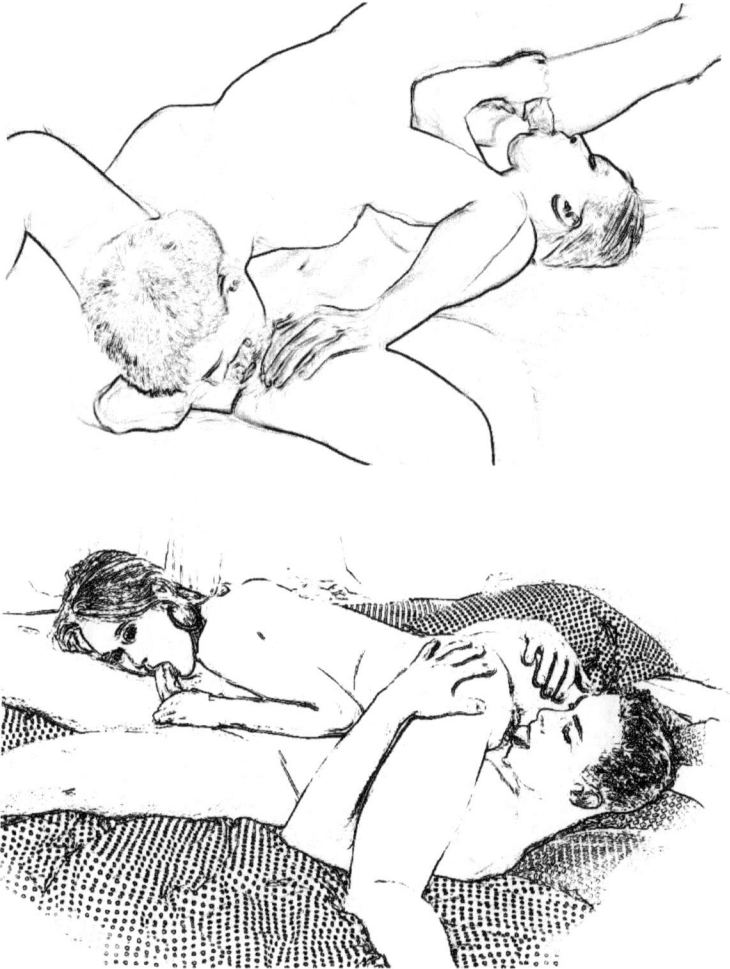

Figure 14. 69 positions

69 positions allow for simultaneous oral sex. You can be on top or bottom, or side-by-side. The 69 position is also used when only one of you is giving oral sex, but it adds a little eroticism by putting the spouse's genitals in the face of the spouse receiving the oral sex. This also stimulates a woman's breasts.

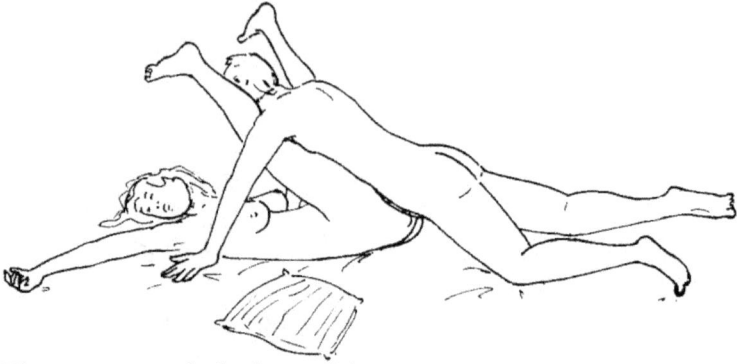

Figure 15. Deckchair position

The Deckchair position involves the wife lying down and putting her legs in the air or on her husband's shoulders.

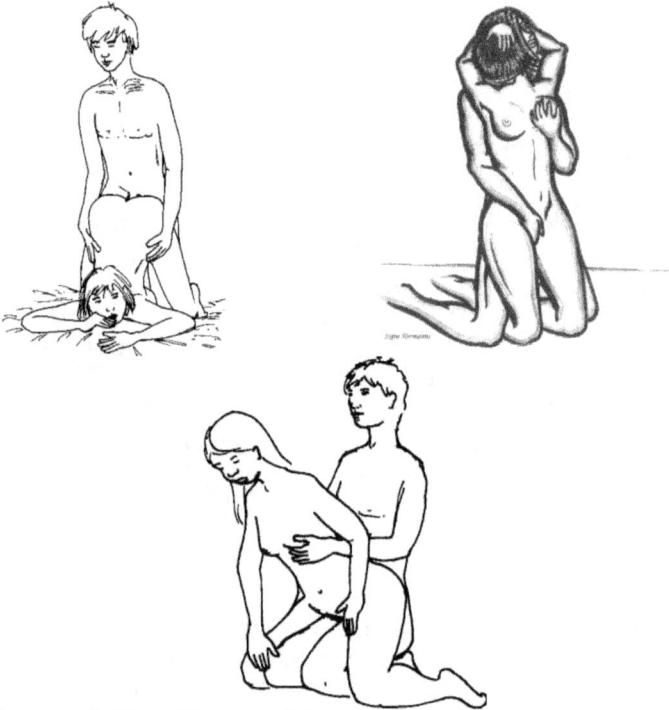

Figure 16. Kneeling positions

Kneeling positions are any that allow one or both spouses to kneel during intercourse.

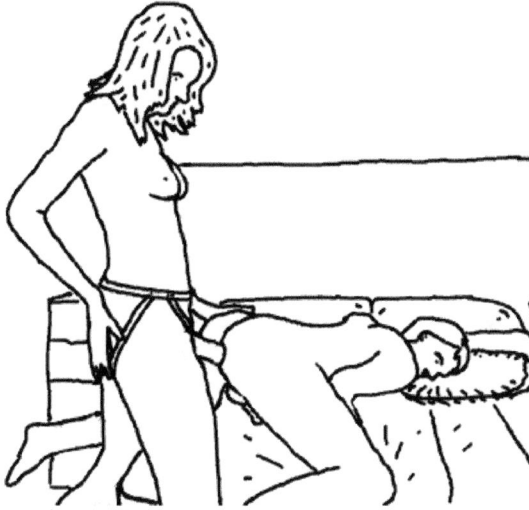

Figure 17. Pegging position

Pegging positions are any that allow the wife to penetrate her husband's anus with a finger or dildo. Figure 17 illustrates a woman using a strap-on dildo so they can fantasize about gender-reversal.

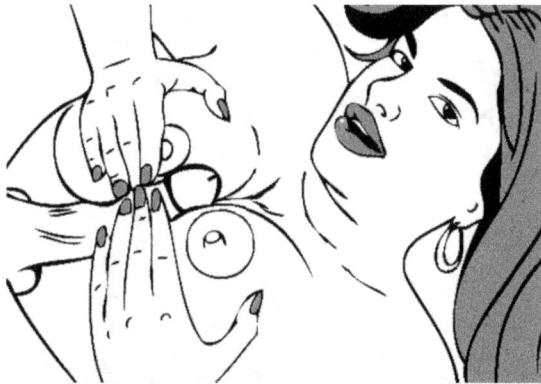

Figure 18. Mammary (Breast) Intercourse Position

Mammary intercourse positions allow the wife to enclose or partially enclose her husband's penis between her breasts. The wife may be lying down with the husband thrusting back and forth, or the husband may be sitting while the wife raises and lowers herself over his penis. An optional technique is for the wife to bend her head down so that the head of the penis enters the wife's mouth.

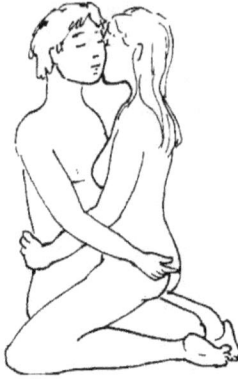

Figure 19. Lotus position

The Lotus position allows the wife to be penetrated while facing her husband and sitting on his lap.

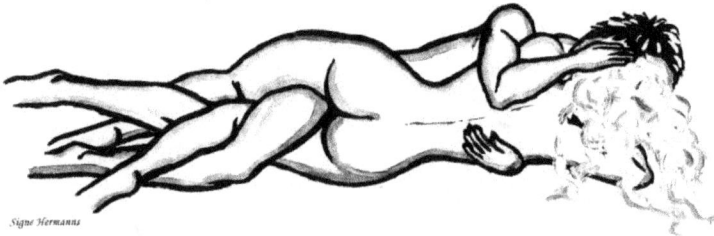

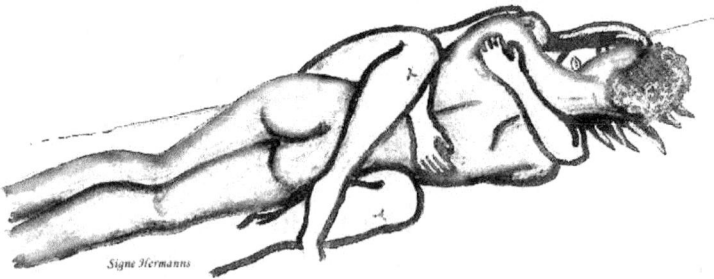

Figure 20. Side-by-side positions

Side-by-side positions allow for intercourse while husband and wife are both lying on their sides.

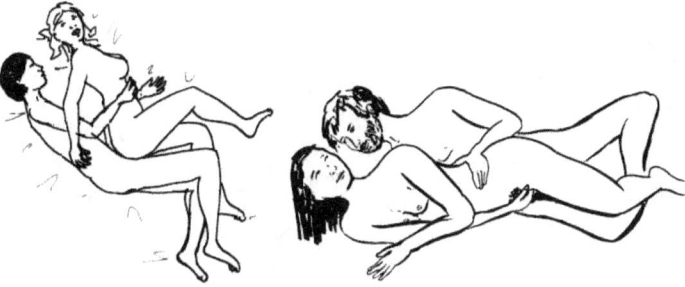

Figure 21. Spooning positions

Spooning positions are those where the husband is facing his wife's back during intercourse, usually while lying down, but sometimes while standing.

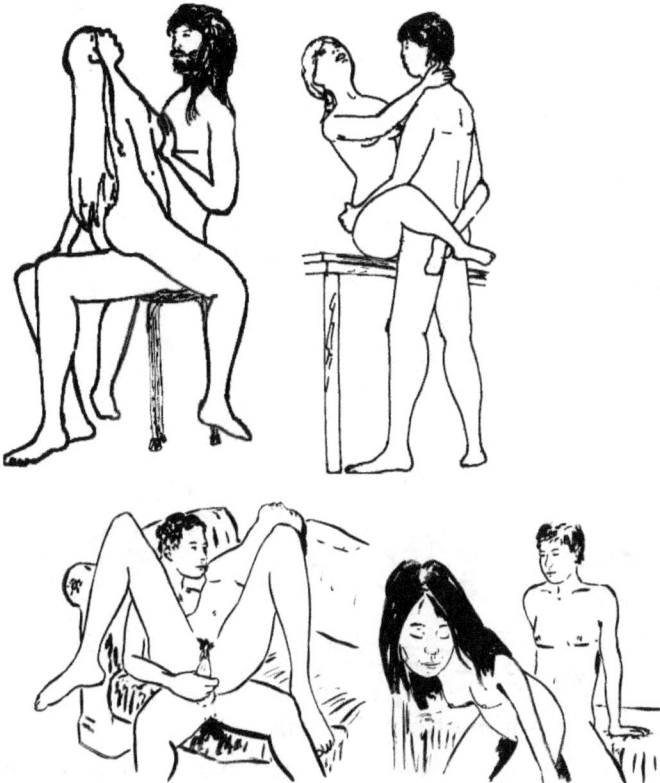

Figure 22. Sitting positions

Sitting positions are any that allow one or both spouses to sit while having intercourse.

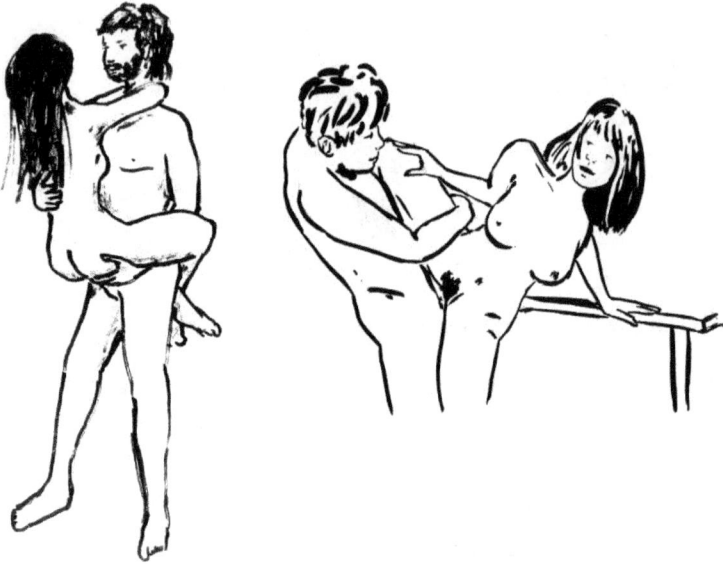

Figure 23. Standing positions

Standing positions involve one or both spouses standing
during intercourse, and may include one or both leaning on
something for support. A stand-and-carry is when the husband
stands with his wife's legs wrapped around his waist during
intercourse.

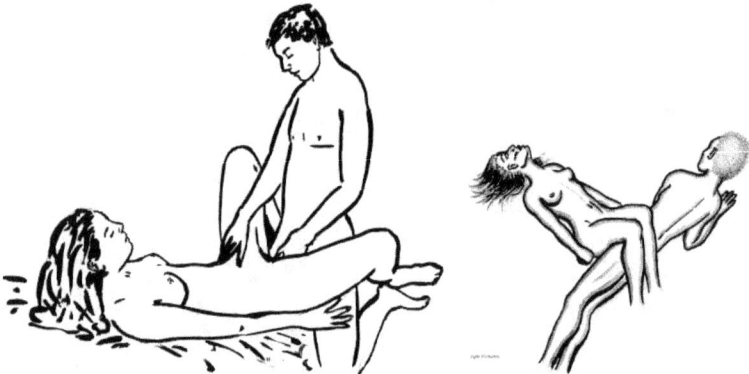

Figure 24. Combination positions

Combination positions involve elements from two or more other
types of positions, such as one lying down while one stands or
kneels.

Pregnancy

Family Planning

You can get married, have sex, have kids, and raise a family as best you can with no real planning. Or, you can plan, in order to try to have a better life than you would without planning.

What does it take to plan a family? Here's one guideline:
1. Decide where you want to live. Which city, which area, what type of home (house, townhouse, mobile home, condo, apartment).
2. Decide what lifestyle you want. Do you want expensive furniture and dinner parties, or will you be happy with average furniture and evenings in front of the TV?
3. Decide how many children you want. Hint: More children costs more money.
4. Estimate how much income you'll need to cover all your costs including your children.
5. Decide if one spouse will stay home full-time or part-time once the first child is born.
6. Establish career plans to reach that income level.

Got all that done? Okay, now you have a plan. Start working to fulfill your plan and save as much as you can toward the day when you'll buy your home or have your first child. When you reach the success point, having bought your house and worked your way up to the salary needed for your family plan, you can ditch the contraception and look forward to all the fun and trials of pregnancy!

Does anyone ever actually do that? A few people do, and they're almost always college graduates.

For the rest of us, we end up with something in the middle. We make some vague plans, work hard without career plans, make some progress, and have our first child before we really intended because our method of contraception failed. But that's okay, we enjoy the pregnancy for the most part, we enjoy our child, we enjoy life. We're an average family, and we're happy.

Getting Pregnant

Pregnancy occurs when one of your husband's sperm merges with one of your ova and the resulting embryo becomes implanted in the lining of your uterus.

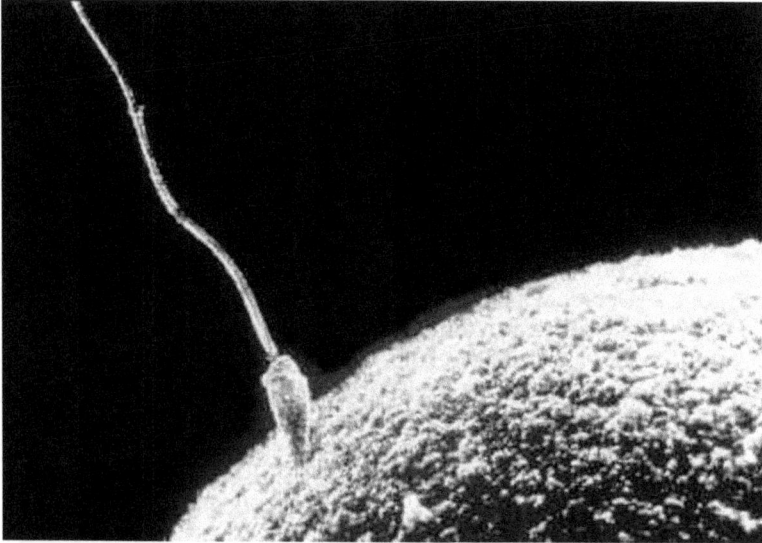

Figure 25. A Sperm About To Fertilize An Ovum.

A normal, healthy woman is fertile (able to become pregnant) for about half of each menstrual cycle. The infertile days are normally those of your period and a few days on either side.

If you want to get pregnant, just have vaginal intercourse as often as possible around the middle of your menstrual cycle. If you have trouble getting pregnant, see a gynecologist or read a book devoted to fertility and pregnancy. There are many things you and your husband can do to increase your fertility, if necessary, and if you have really serious problems, it may be possible for doctors to harvest one of your ova and fertilize it with one of your husband's sperm in a laboratory, then implant it in your uterus.

If you don't want to get pregnant, then either don't have sex, or use one or more methods of contraception when you have sex. Almost everybody wants to have sex, of course, so the next section presents your options for contraception.

Contraception

Is contraception okay for Christians? Some people believe that contraception is sinful, and that sex should only be performed when you want to have a baby. The Catholic Church leaders are famous for that belief. However, their position had to be reasoned out, because that policy is not in the Bible. Grandma Synthia strongly disagrees with that reasoning, primarily because it denies human nature.

There is a sinful nature that Godly people should resist, but a normal sex drive is *not* part of a sinful nature, it's part of God's design. The sinful nature is what temps us to steal or lie. God gave us sex, and he gave us libidos that periodically demand sexual satisfaction. Trying to deny that hunger is like trying to not drink when you're thirsty – you can do it for awhile, but it gets harder and harder, and it's not necessary in order to be Godly. On the contrary, give thanks to God when you have water to drink when you're thirsty, and give thanks to God when you can satisfy your sex drive with your spouse while using a contraceptive method to avoid pregnancy when you're not prepared for pregnancy!

If you agree that contraception is okay, then you have a lot of options. You and your husband, or husband-to-be if you're about to get married, need to discuss these options and decide which ones you're going to try.

Notice we said "*try*", because most methods of contraception have significant failure rates. For that reason, you may want to consider using more than one, and if you have an unplanned pregnancy, you might try different ones.

The goal of contraception is to prevent sperm from getting to your ova by blocking the sperm, killing the sperm, preventing your body from releasing ova, or preventing a fertilized ovum from implanting in your uterus.

Birth Control Pills

When you become pregnant, your body changes the levels of many hormones, and some of those changes make your body stop releasing ova. That's why a pregnant woman can't get pregnant with a second child while she's already pregnant.

Birth control pills are designed to artificially adjust your hormones to imitate hormones at pregnancy levels, in order to stop your ovaries from releasing ova. No ova, no pregnancy.

You need to see a doctor to get prescription for birth control pills, and it will cost about $15-30 per month.

Breastfeeding

Breastfeeding reduces the likelihood of pregnancy, and is free, but is highly unreliable.

Condoms

Condoms are penis-shaped balloons made of latex or some other material, and are designed to cover your husband's penis and capture all his semen so it can't get inside you. If a condom breaks while you're having vaginal intercourse, almost all of it gets inside you, and it's like you didn't use a condom at all. The failure rate is usually between 5 and 10 percent of the time, so if you rely on condoms alone, odds are pretty high that you're going to get pregnant sooner or later.

An advantage of condoms is that, if you or your husband became infected with a sexually transmitted disease before you got married, they can prevent the transfer of STDs between you. But again, if the condom breaks, it's just like you didn't use one at all.

A disadvantage of condoms is that they decrease the physical sensation, and therefore the pleasure, that men experience.

> **Obsolete Sex Tip:** Great-Great-Grandma Theodora taught Grandma Flora how to make condoms from sheep or pig intestines, and treat them with lye. For some reason, Grandma Flora didn't pass that particular knowledge on to her granddaughters...

Condoms cost anywhere from 35 cents to $2 each, depending on brand and quantity. Condoms can be washed and reused with little degradation, but with a failure rate as high as 10% for brand new ones, you might want to think twice about recycling them. Many county health departments will give you a big bag of them for free.

Diaphragms and Cervical Caps (Shields)

The diaphragm is a soft latex or silicone dome with a spring molded into the rim, and the spring creates a seal against the walls of the vagina to prevent semen from reaching the cervix. A spermicide is usually used to increase effectiveness and make it easier to insert. The diaphragm must be inserted into the vagina before sexual intercourse, and remain in place for 6 to 8 hours after a man's last ejaculation.

Diaphragms come in different sizes, and must be fitted by a professional. Diaphragms should be re-fitted after a weight change of 10 lbs or more, and after a pregnancy. Also, a separate diaphragm of a different size is needed during your period.

A prescription is required in the United States, and they cost anywhere from $15-60 each.

Cervical caps are similar to diaphragms except they are smaller and made to fit only over the cervix. They also have to be custom fitted by a professional.

IUDs

An intra-uterine device (IUD) is an simple object that a doctor places into your uterus and usually has a part that hangs down into the cervical opening between the uterus and vagina. Despite the fact that no one understands how these things prevent pregnancy, they have a very high success rate, 97-99%, and work until you have a doctor remove it.

An IUD costs $250 or more, plus the doctor's fees, but last up to 10 years and don't monkey around with your hormones.

Masturbation

Masturbation is where you, your husband, or both of you manipulate yourselves to achieve orgasms. As long as his sperm don't get to your vagina, this is completely effective.

Be careful, though, because a single drop of semen can contain literally millions of sperm, and if a drop gets to moisture near your labia, that might be enough for some of them to swim all the way inside. The odds may be against it, but it only takes 1 to make a baby.

Physically, masturbation is very easy, but some people struggle with the mental and emotional aspects of masturbating in front of their spouse, and some people object to it for spiritual reasons. Later in this book, an entire chapter is devoted to the topic of masturbation.

Masturbation is free and convenient.

Morning-After Pills

Morning-after pills are so named because they're taken the day or two after you had sex without contraception. They may prevent a sperm from fertilizing your ovum, or they may prevent a fertilized ovum from implanting in your uterus.

We couldn't find any reliable information on how often a failure-to-implant occurs naturally, but it is clear that it does happen. Many people believe that preventing a fertilized ovum from implanting is a form of abortion, rather than a form of birth control, but Grandma Synthia sees this as replicating a natural event, similar to using birth control pills to replicate the way your body naturally prevents the release of ova while you're pregnant.

The failure rate is a little more complicated than that of something like a condom, because a condom works unless it tears or gets pulled off inside the vagina. A morning-after pill, however, can only be effective if you would have otherwise gotten pregnant. With that taken into consideration, the manufacturers estimate a success rate of 80-90%.

The primary morning-after drugs are mifepristone and levonorgestrel. Mifepristone can be used as a morning-after medication or in higher doses it can cause an abortion of an established pregnancy. Levonorgestrel, marketed as Plan B®, can only work as a morning-after pill, because it can't abort an existing pregnancy.

Plan B® is available in most pharmacies without a prescription, for about $50. **WARNING:** To date, the only safety studies we have found have been with small numbers of women, who only used it one time, and they were only monitored for short periods of time. We found no studies on the long term effects, or on the effects for repeated use, or for women with specific characteristics that might cause complications. These medications have the potential to cause problems if only used a single time, and it's possible that repeated use could increase the likelihood or severity of complications.

Non-Vaginal Intercourse

Oral, breast, and anal sex all provide options for your husband to experience an intercourse-based orgasm without risking pregnancy. It is completely effective as long as you're careful not to get any of the semen near your labia.

Spermicide

Spermicide is a chemical you put in your vagina before intercourse, and it's designed to kill any sperm before they get through to your uterus. It has a high failure rate when used alone, so it's usually used with condoms, diaphragms, cervical caps, or sponges.

Spermicides are unscented, clear, unflavored, non-staining, and provide vaginal lubrication. It costs about $1-2 per use.

Sponges

Contraceptive sponges are usually contain spermicide and are inserted into the vagina just prior to intercourse and placed in front of the cervix, to both block and kill sperm.

Effectiveness ranges from 68-99%, depending on placement, and cost $2-3 per spermicide-soaked sponge. They may be used with condoms to increase overall effectiveness.

Timing

Timing methods such as the Rhythm method, Standard Days Method, or various methods of fertility monitoring are intended to help you determine when you are fertile. Then you have sexual intercourse without other contraceptive methods only on your infertile days. On your fertile days you either abstain from sex or use other means of contraception.

Warning: While it is unlikely that you will get pregnant if you have sex immediately before, during, or immediately after your period, *it is possible*. If you're not ready for pregnancy financially, emotionally, or in any other way, do not depend on timing alone to prevent pregnancy.

Tubal Ligation

Tubal ligation (getting your "tubes tied") is surgery to permanently sterilize a woman by cutting her fallopian tubes to prevent ova from reaching the uterus or sperm. The reliability is near, but not quite, 100%.

Hormone production, libido, and the menstrual cycle can all be affected by tubal ligation. There is now a high success rate for reversing tubal ligation, but it is also major surgery.

Tubal Ligation vs. Vasectomy

If you and your husband have decided that you want a permanent solution to prevent pregnancy, a vasectomy is far better for 2 major reasons.

First, because the vas deferends are in a man's scrotum, a vasectomy is minor surgery, whereas the location of a woman's fallopian tubes deep inside her abdomen make tubal ligation a much riskier major surgery.

Second, a vasectomy will have no impact on a man's hormones or libido, while tubal ligation can have a major impact on both a woman's hormones and her libido.

Vaginal Ring

Vaginal rings are used to slowly release hormones to have an effect like birth control pills. Rings are easily inserted and removed, and are left in place for 3 weeks, then removed for 1 week to allow for a period to occur. Vaginal walls hold them in place near the cervix, but their exact location is not important. Most couples report no interference or discomfort, and many cannot feel the ring at all during intercourse.

Marketed under the name "NuvaRing", you use you 1 ring per month at a cost of about $65 per ring.

Vasectomy

A minor surgical procedure in which a man is sterilized by cutting the two vas deferends in the scrotum. This prevents sperm from getting into his semen, but does not affect a man's sexual desire or ability. He can still get aroused, have normal erections, and ejaculate semen. The only difference is that the semen contains no sperm.

Reliability is almost, but not quite, 100%. Vasectomies are permanent and normally irreversible.

Warning: Do not have a vasectomy with the expectation that it can be reversed. While it possible, success rates are barely above 50%, are often temporary, and significantly increase the rate of birth defects.

Withdrawal

Also known by the Latin term *coitus interruptus*, this method has you and your husband having vaginal intercourse on your fertile days, but he withdraws before he has an orgasm inside you.

It is possible for a husband to pull out just as he begins to have an orgasm, but this increases the risk that some semen will make it into the vagina. More commonly, either you or your husband would use your hands to finish getting him to orgasm. Alternatively, he could finish in your mouth or anus, in a toy vagina, or not finish at all.

Warning: Your husband can be releasing sperm inside you even before he reaches orgasm. The relatively small numbers of sperm you get this way are not likely to get you pregnant, but they may. The fact is, it only takes one. In addition, if he spews his sperm outside your vagina, you should be careful that it's not near your vagina. Sperm swim, and if any semen reaches the moisture in or around your vagina, they can swim all the way inside you.

Contraceptive Myths

Douching

Douching with any substance immediately following intercourse will *not* prevent pregnancy.

While it may seem reasonable to try to wash the semen out of the vagina, douching actually spreads semen further towards the uterus. Even if that were not the case, you wouldn't be able to douche fast enough, as millions of sperm will swim into your uterus within seconds of your husband's ejaculation inside your vagina.

Urination

Urinating after sex does *not* prevent pregnancy. It is advised to help prevent urinary tract infections, but it will not get any sperm out of your vagina, nor will it kill any sperm in your vagina.

Unplanned Pregnancy

If you do get pregnant when you didn't plan to, you have 3 options:

1. Give birth to the baby and raise it as well as you can despite the lack of preparation.
2. Give birth and give the baby up for adoption.
3. Have an abortion to kill the baby.

Your emotions may be very strong and very volatile if you learn that you're pregnant and you didn't intend to be. Women usually avoid pregnancy because they're having casual sex with someone they don't expect to marry, they're having sex before marriage, they're having sex within marriage but they don't have time to care for a baby, or because they can't afford the expenses of a baby. Any of those situations could justify strong emotions, if not outright panic.

Well, Grandma isn't the one who's pregnant, so she's not upset, and this advice is intended to be objective and practical.

First, forget having an abortion. Yes, you have a right to control your body, but a baby is a *separate* body of another human being inside your body. The fetus is not *your* body. Different DNA – different body, even though it's inside your body. You had sex and now you're pregnant and upset. Tough. Make plans for carrying your baby to term over the next nine months, and start working on the decision of keeping your baby versus giving your baby up for adoption.

This book is intended primarily for women who are married or are about to be, but if you're single and reading this, here's a complicated set of rules to determine whether to give up your baby, or keep it. Because it's so complicated, we're going to number the steps to help you keep them straight:

1. You're single, so give your baby up for adoption.

Well, maybe that wasn't so complicated. When you're pregnant, the only responsible thing to do is whatever is best for the *baby*. If you're single, unless you're independently wealthy, you can't afford to take care of your baby properly. Oh, sure, you can imagine 1,000 ways of working it out so you can keep your baby, and 900 of them are variations of getting your Mom to babysit, and getting your Dad to give you money in emergencies (which will be all the time). All of which is to serve *your* desire to keep your baby, not what's in the best interest of your baby. Love your baby enough to do what's very hard for you but what's best for your baby: give it up for adoption.

If you're married and have an unplanned pregnancy, your choices can be affected by your family income. If you and your husband are barely earning above minimum wage, living in a tiny old mobile home, and wondering how you'll fix your car the next time it breaks down, you have no real choice if you love your child: You must give it up for adoption because its what's best for your child. You can't afford a baby.

If you and your husband are doing at least a little bit better than barely scraping by, then you have a real choice. If you keep your baby, it will cost a lot of money, so if your income does not go up, your standard of living must go down. Every $100 you spend on diapers, clothes, or doctor visits is $100 you can't spend on anything else. You'll have to eat cheaper, dress cheaper, driver cheaper cars, skip buying a new TV, spend less on college tuition, live in a smaller house or apartment, or all of the above.

If you and your husband both graduated from college long ago, have high paying careers, a big house, fancy cars, and eat out at classy restaurants frequently, guess what? You can afford a baby. You'll still have to lower your standard of living a little bit, but not by as much, percentage-wise. For you, it's only a matter of whether you *want* to keep your baby.

Think of it this way. If a baby costs $3000 worth of expenses in its first year, what percentage of your family income is that? If you and your husband earn $30,000, your baby will lower your standard of living by 10%. If your family income is $120,000, then your baby will only lower your standard of living 2.5%. In the first case, you take sack lunches to work every day, work as much overtime as possible, and fix the car yourself. In the second case, you simply postpone trading in one of your cars for an extra year, and your 3% annual raise will put you right back where you were before you had the baby.

Abortion

Yes, you have a right to control your body, but a baby is a *separate* body of another human being inside your body, it's not *your* body. Every cell that is part of your body has the same DNA that you've had since you father's sperm fertilized your mother's egg. From the time that your egg is fertilized by a sperm, your baby's DNA is different from yours. It is alive, it is human, and its DNA proves that it is not part of your body. Don't be pressured into an abortion by anyone, especially a boyfriend.

Likely disadvantages of abortion:
- Anger
- Anxiety
- Guilt
- Regret

Possible disadvantages of abortion:
- Adverse effects on sexual functions
- Clinical depression
- Death
- Post Abortion Syndrome (PAS)
- Post-surgical pain
- Severe blood loss
- Sterility
- Suicidal behaviors

Advantages of abortion:
- You kill off a baby you don't want, so you don't have to be bothered by it.
- If you're single and you kill your baby quickly enough, your parents might not find out you had sex.
- An abortion is cheaper than the hospital and doctor fees if you don't have insurance. You may save *hundreds* of dollars by killing your baby.

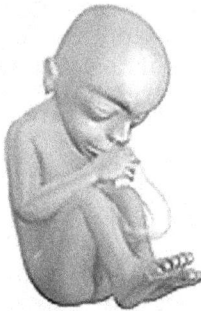

Figure 26. Your baby at 20 weeks.

What's Wrong With Sex?

Normal Limits

There are restrictions on the circumstances of sex that vary with nations and religions. Grandma Anne is an American and a Protestant Christian, so this advice reflects that, and restrictions include who, what, when, where, and how. Fortunately, Grandma's restrictions are all very simple...

Who: Have sex only with your husband.
What: Your husband can't be an animal.
When: Only have sex after you get married.
Where: Anywhere that's just the two of you.
How: Husband and wife must both agree, every time.

Some folks also think there are restrictions regarding **why**, but Grandma doesn't. Usually these objections are that sex should only be for the purpose of creating children. Grandma's immediate response to that idea is, "phooey". For a more detailed response, read the next chapter, What's Right With Sex.

A lot of people have a lot of ideas about restrictions regarding sex, many of them with no reasons, and most of the rest with bad reasons. Grandma has a principle for determining what's okay regarding sex, and what's not, and here it is:

**There must be a specific reason for
prohibiting or limiting a sexual activity,
or it's okay.**

Well, Grandma has already listed the restrictions, so now let's explain the main reasons...

Who: Having sex only between a husband and wife eliminates all sexual diseases. That's reason enough. That's right, if a man and woman never have sex with anyone other than their spouse, they cannot have a sexually transmitted disease. True, you can get a "sexually transmitted disease" such as HIV through blood transfusions of tainted blood, but that's not actually transmitted to the victim by sex, is it? And blood can only be tainted if its donated by someone who has a sexual disease because they had sex with someone other than their spouse. So sex only inside marriage is beneficial to the community as well as each couple.

In addition, the Bible makes it very clear that only a husband and wife should have sex. Having sex with anyone else damages a relationship permanently. It often destroys marriages, but even if a marriage survives infidelity, and some level of trust is restored, most cheated spouses will never be able to trust their spouse as much as they did before. That makes the relationship less than it could and should be.

Even if one spouse doesn't know the other committed adultery, it can affect the attitude of the spouse who committed adultery and it can have an impact on the relationship in many subtle ways.

What: Only have sex with a human. If you abide by the rule of having sex only with your husband or wife, you've got this one covered.

Also, Grandma Elizabeth found a non-religious reason to prohibit bestiality: it may be a means of viruses crossing the species barrier. How would you like to have sex with an animal, get a virus from it, have that virus mutate inside you, and then you pass it on to a human partner?

For Christians and most other major religions, the restriction is loud and clear, never have sex with an animal. Period.

When: Only have sex after you get married, because the rule of having sex only with your husband or wife requires a marriage first.

When you should get married is a different issue, as far as legal age limits, parents' permission, preparedness for a permanent commitment, and readiness to start a family, but as far as sex is concerned, wait until you're married.

Where: Anywhere that's just the two of you if you don't want to be embarrassed. There are no national or state governments that Grandma Elizabeth could find that legally allow having sex in public. All major religions other than humanism prohibit having sex in public, and most humanists seem to concur with this principle.

There are private sex clubs where it is legal to have sex in front of other people, and others where it is tolerated, and you can put a video or live-stream of yourselves on the Internet, but the only way to guarantee that your friends and family can't see you is not to participate in these ventures.

How: Husband and wife must both agree, every time. The only way to have sexual intercourse without consent is by force, and that's rape.

If you and your husband both agree to have sex, then you can be sure that God approves of your sexual activity.

But What's God doing while I'm having sex?
Can you be holy while having sex? Well, can you be holy while eating lunch? The answer to both is yes!

If you're having sex with your husband in private and you both consent, it's holy, because those are the only restrictions he put on it. In fact, the overly restrained should think about this: Not having sex can be unholy. Yes, that's right, if your spouse needs sexual release in an orgasm, or just emotional closeness from sex without orgasm, and you withhold it, you are harming your spouse, and *that* is unholy.

God designed men and women to have sex. He's not surprised by it, and he's not embarrassed by it.

You can eat food without enjoying it, but food has taste so that we can enjoy it! Similarly, God designed us to enjoy sex and the pleasure of orgasms. Why would you turn down a gift that God Himself has given you?

Think of it this way: God takes joy in our joy. So if you refrain from the joy of sex without a good reason, you're denying God the pleasure He would otherwise derive from your pleasure. The pleasure that He intended for you to have.

Abnormal Sex

Abnormal sex is sexual behavior in one of these categories:
- Dangerous
- Compulsive
- Excessive to the point of harmfully limiting normal life activities.

Medically, there is no such thing as an addition to sex or to pornography. An **addiction** is a physical dependence on a non-nutritive chemical to the point where the chemical is required for normal functioning. Such dependence is associated with constant cravings, preoccupation with obtaining the chemical, decreased motivation for normal life activities, and with many chemicals, intoxication. What is commonly referred to as sexual addiction is covered under the compulsive and excessive types of sexual behavior.

Dangerous Sexual Behavior

Dangerous sex is sexual behavior with a high risk of serious disease or that can cause serious physical or psychological harm.

Disease

There are numerous sexually transmitted diseases (STDs),[7] the worst of which, at the time of this writing, is the HIV virus, which can result in AIDS, and is life-threatening. Some STDs can be cured with medical treatment, and symptoms from most of the rest can be improved with medical treatment.

If you do not have an STD, the more partners you have sex with, the higher the odds that you will contract an STD.

If you do have an STD, the more partners you have sex with, the higher the odds that you will contract an additional STD, and the higher the odds that you will infect other people. If you are married, adultery increases the risks of disease to you and your spouse.

The only certain way to avoid all sexually transmitted diseases is to marry a virgin and never be sexually intimate with anyone other than your spouse.

---

[7] Also known as Sexually Transmitted Infection (STI).

Condoms can significantly reduce the risk of infection from sexual diseases, but cannot eliminate the risk. Condoms may prevent infection in a single sexual encounter, but over many encounters they may simply delay when infection first occurs. Because condoms are only about 90% effective, 100 encounters means about 10 encounters with a failed condom. The only way to eliminate the risk is to not have sex with an infected person.

The only way to be sure your sexual partner does not have a sexual disease is if they have never been sexually intimate (including kissing and oral sex), or if they have not been sexually intimate since they were tested for every STD and found to be negative. If a person has been sexually intimate even once since they were tested, even if they used a condom in that encounter, they could now be infected. And this assumes the tests were not false-negative and that the person does not have some new STD that tests are not being conducted for.[8]

If a person tells you they are a virgin and they are not, they may infect you.

If a person tells you they do not have an STD and they are lying or they are wrong, they may infect you.

If you have an STD, it is your moral responsibility to tell anyone you may become sexually intimate with *before* you are sexually intimate.

If you have an STD and want to find a partner with the same STD so that you cannot infect one another, seek a support group that offers dating services.

If you wish to avoid or limit risky sexual behavior, you can seek psychological help from physicians or support groups.

Physical Harm

The forms of sexual behavior that can cause serious physical harm are primarily sadomasochism and bondage.

Sadism refers to inflicting pain or humiliation upon another person, and masochism refers to inflicting pain or humiliation upon yourself. Put another way, sadists enjoy inflicting pain,

---

[8] HIV was being transmitted for years before the medical community became aware of it, developed screening tests, and began routine testing.

and masochists enjoy receiving pain. Sadomasochism is also known as S&M.

It is certainly possible to engage in sadomasochism and cause temporary pain, without causing serious physical harm. The danger is often one of care or degree. For example, light spanking may merely sting, while a harder strike may break a bone or put out an eye.

Many sadomasochists establish safe-words as codes to stop. Part of typical activity for a masochist is crying and begging the sadist to stop, when they don't really want them to stop. The safe-word is a term that they would not normally use, to signal to the sadist that the masochist really does want them to stop. The danger here is if one of the parties forgets the safe-word, or if the sadist gets carried away and is slow to recognize it.

Bondage, also known as bondage and discipline (BD), involves people being physically restrained, such as being tied up, gagged, or blindfolded.

Real bondage should not be confused with play bondage. In play bondage, a person is not actually tied up, and can easily get themselves out of their sham restraints.

While real bondage can be performed without causing serious physical harm, it involves real restraints from which the subject cannot free themselves. It often involves tying the subject into particular bodily positions or suspending them in the air. The dangers here include restricted blood flow, restricted air flow, damage from hyper-extended joints, damage from over-stressed joints, and the subject remaining bound too long should the dominant person become incapacitated.

Although sadomasochism and bondage are distinct and can be practiced distinctly, they are often engaged in simultaneously, and that is known as BDSM.

If you can't enjoy sex without participating in such risky sexual behavior, you should seek psychological help from physicians or support groups.

Compulsive Sexual Behavior

A compulsion is a behavior which a person does because they feel they must, not because they enjoy it. Sexual compulsion is referred to as hypersexuality, and was previously known as nymphomania, furor uterinus, and satyriasis.

Hypersexuality is an abnormal need for frequent genital stimulation to the point that it interferes with normal life activities, and the genital stimulation usually provides no satisfaction, and can have physiological and neurological symptoms.

Hypersexuality is not enjoyable, and worse, it may be dangerous by causing the person to have sex with many different partners in a vain attempt to satisfy irresistible sexual urges.

Hypersexuality is a serious malady and can be caused by cancer, adrenal malfunctions, bipolar disorder, and other diseases. If you or your spouse ever develop hypersexuality symptoms, you should seek immediate medical help.

Excessive Sexual Behavior

In contrast to addictions, risky behavior, and compulsions, harmful excess is a failure to safely limit a behavior which a person enjoys and which causes no ill effects in moderation, but can cause serious problems in excess. Non-sexual examples are non-compulsive overeating, overspending, and out-of-control gambling.

While a person may consider their spouse's sexual interests or libido to be excessive if greater than their own, it's only abnormal if it is excessive to the point of harmfully limiting normal life activities.

For example, a husband may enjoy viewing pornographic pictures over the Internet. If he typically spends 20 minutes in this activity once every few days, it's not abnormal behavior if he enjoys it and it's not harmfully limiting his life activities. At the other end of the spectrum, however, if a husband stops going to work and spends every waking hour viewing pornography, that is abnormal because it's interfering with normal life activities.

For excessive sexual behavior, the primary symptoms include spending excessive time in sexual activities, spending excessive amounts of money in sexual activities, pursuit of many sexual partners, escalation to dangerous behavior, or serious disagreement with a spouse.[9]

Determining what is excessive can be subjective, and dealing with it can be difficult. Like the excessive behaviors of overeating, overspending, and problem gambling, it can have a major impact on the spouse, and the assistance a spouse can provide can be quite limited.

Disagreement with a spouse can be a particularly difficult subject. For example, a husband's masturbation might be the subject of disagreement between the husband and his wife. If the husband satisfies his libido through masturbation alone, and forsakes his responsibilities to help his wife be sexually fulfilled, that is excessive behavior on the husband's part, and the marital disagreement may be his fault. However, if the wife refuses to participate in sex with her husband often enough to meet his needs, he masturbates for relief when she is not available or willing, and she objects to that, then the disagreement might be primarily her fault.

If a person with an excessive sexual behavior recognizes that they have a problem and wants to do something about it, one of the best solutions is a 12-step recovery program. The American Psychological Association summarizes the 12-step approach as involving the following points:[10]

- Admitting that one cannot control one's addiction or compulsion.
- Recognizing a greater power that can give strength.
- Examining past errors with the help of a sponsor (experienced member).
- Making amends for these errors.
- Learning to live a new life with a new code of behavior.
- Helping others that suffer from the same addictions or compulsions.

---

[9] In the New Testament, the English word for excessive sexual behavior is lasciviousness, which is translated from the Greek word aselgeia, and is not the same as lust, which comes from the Greek word epithumeo. For more about lust, see the chapter on Fantasy vs. Lust.

[10] VandenBos, Gary R. (2007). APA dictionary of psychology, 1st edition, Washington, DC: American Psychological Association.

Note that for some excessive behaviors, complete avoidance of the behavior might be best, such as with problem gambling, but for other issues like overeating, complete abstinence is not possible. Excessive sexual behavior may be of either kind, in that it might be possible to avoid all pornography, but it is extremely difficult to completely suppress a healthy libido.

God designed men and women to have sex.

He's not surprised by it, and he's not embarrassed by it.

WHAT'S RIGHT WITH SEX?

The Advantages Of Sex

Sex is great! It has all these advantages and more:

Procreation: The first and best way to make a baby! Although it's now possible for doctors to fertilize a woman's egg with her husband's sperm in a laboratory, sex is easier, faster, less expensive, and more fun for a healthy husband and wife.

Pleasure: Before, during, and after orgasm, nothing else provides so much physical pleasure from so little effort.

Intimate Relationship-Building: Having a sexual relationship with someone does not *require* emotional intimacy, but it is an *opportunity* for emotional intimacy better than any other.

Exercise: Movement is exercise, and you cannot have sex without movement. The human body is designed to move, and it generally it takes a lot of movement and a fast heartbeat to get to an orgasm.

Fun and Recreation: Oh, wow, for a healthy couple with a healthy relationship, sex is fun, fun, fun! It requires no expensive equipment, no membership fees, no special training, no travel, no special clothes (no clothes!). *Although some of those can add to the fun.*

Pain-Relief: Sexual arousal causes your brain to create endorphin hormones which can override pain-processing in the brain.

Anti-Depressant: Sex can be a powerful way to relieve a depressed mood and help avoid a decline into something more severe. And it can sometimes provide a positive effect in relief of clinical depression (major depressive disorders), depending on the type and cause of the depression.

Stress-Reduction: Emotional stresses are cumulative and long-lasting, and even happy events such as marriages and births are stressful.[11] Healthy sexual activity helps counter the effects of stress by the physical exercise and emotional comfort.

Motivation: Sort of the flip-side of countering depression, sex can also be excellent in providing inspiration and enthusiasm for life. By that, we don't mean one spouse promising to have sex if the other spouse does something for them, which you should never do. No, we mean that a healthy sexual relationship, without unduly frustrated sex drives, can help people derive enough enjoyment that it gives them a positive outlook on life.

The Principle Of Godly Sex

What kinds of sexual activities are okay between a husband and wife? Every kind that both agree to.

**Every kind of sexual activity between
a husband and wife that both
of them agree to is okay!**

Every kind between a husband and wife that both of them agree to. Think about your questions, your wildest questions, about what kind of conduct is okay. What about... this kind, that kind, oh, the really, really raunchy, dirty, low-class, unmentionable kind like... The answer is *every* kind.

There is nothing you and your husband can do regarding sexual activity that is wrong if you both agree. That means physically, and in your *minds*!

For many readers, that may raise a lot of doubts, and we'll try to address all doubts one at a time throughout this book, starting with *the* most common doubt, that of sexual fantasies. That's covered in the very next chapter.

---

[11] See the Holmes and Rahe Stress Scale for more information (also known as Life Events Stress Test, Life Events Scale, or Social Readjustment Rating Scale).

Now, you may have noticed, along with highly experienced Bible scholars, that the Bible does not explicitly say that it's okay to have sex on a living room sofa. Does that mean it's wrong to have sex on a living room sofa? No, of course not. The Bible is not a sex manual, and it not a catalog of every possible sexual activity with a check mark in a column for okay or not okay.

The Bible also does not say that you must be on a bed to have sex. Neither does the Bible tell you how many times a day to brush your teeth. We're not trying to be irreverent here, we're trying to make a point. The Bible gives us some rules for life, such as *do not steal*, but it also gives us principles. **For life not covered by specific rules, we are to figure out how to live based on the principles.** Other than a few specific rules, sexual activity must all be based on principles.

> The primary principle for Godly sex is that husbands and wives should satisfy each other's sex drives and that the only restrictions are to have sexual intercourse only with your spouse, only when you both agree, and not to desire sex with anyone other than your spouse.
> Therefore, everything other than those restrictions is permissible in a Godly life.

This principle means it's okay to enjoy sex, including oral sex, anal sex, masturbation, and sexual fantasies (which is not the same as lust). It's okay to have foreplay or intercourse for many hours, or for only a few minutes as long as both the husband's and wife's sexual needs are being met.

Wives being sexually assertive is okay. It's not only okay, it's *required* to fully satisfy your husband's emotional needs. Assertive sex acts can be a minor part of your sex life, but it is an essential part of a full sex life for a woman, because it's how you show your husband a positive desire. It is the critical difference between being *willing* to have sex, and *wanting* to have sex, and the difference to your husband is extremely important.

The essence of Grandma's sex advice to young brides is built around two principles: It's okay for a wife to enjoy sex, and it's important a wife to keep her husband satisfied sexually. Many young Christian women seem to intuitively agree with the second, but have trouble with the first. That's a problem, however, because you can't do your best at keeping your husband satisfied if you don't enjoy sex. Why? Again, it's the difference between *willing* and *wanting*.

You may be willing to have sex any time your husband asks for it, but that alone puts too much pressure on him – if he always has to initiate sex, it can lead him to feel like he's imposing, which in turn, leads him to be reluctant to ask. If he always or usually gets sex when he asks for it, it will relieve his physical hunger, but *having a wife who <u>wants</u> to have sex with him will meet his <u>emotional</u> needs and boost his self-esteem like nothing else can.*

Sex is a wonderful part of God's design, and a natural desire for mentally and physically healthy men and women. So, most of Grandma's sex advice focuses on why and how to enjoy sex yourself, and how to be a vixen in the bedroom to help your husband be all he can be.

FANTASY VS. LUST

- The Problem
- The Biblical Meaning of Lust
- Thinking About Sex
- Sexual Fantasy
- Fantasy In God's Design

The Problem

It's common knowledge:

> Most Christians struggle with sex.

Ask any group of teenage or adult Christians, "Do Christians struggle with sex?", and the answer will be a nearly unanimous "Yes." And it's not just Christians, but most religious people. Pretty much everyone who believes that humans are more than mere animals, and even some people who think that humans are nothing more than a lucky species that evolved.

Except that the first statement above is phrased wrong. Most people don't struggle with sex. That is, most people don't have to struggle to have physical sex. What they struggle with are sexual thoughts.

Okay, now that we've pointed out that difference, everyone will say, "of course, that's what we meant." But that wasn't the statement. Why do people hear "struggles with sex" and subconsciously think "struggles with sexual thoughts"?

Well, perhaps because when we have difficulty struggling with sexual thoughts, we try to avoid or minimize sexual thoughts. Sure, we know it's okay to have sexual thoughts about our spouse, but any sexual thoughts beyond that is either wrong, might be wrong, or might lead into thoughts that are wrong. So we become reluctant to think about sex, and one of the repercussions of that reluctance to think about sexual things may be to avoid thinking about the process and nature of thinking about sex. And as a result, we use intuitive notions and common knowledge instead of examining the issues carefully.

What do we base our expectations on regarding sexual thoughts? Generally they seem to be based on the belief that lust is sinful[12] and some variation of one of these two ideas:

- **x**   Lust is sexual desire.
- **x**   Lust is thinking about sex.

Wikipedia, the people's encyclopedia, defines "lust" as *any intense desire or craving for gratification and excitement.*[13] That seems to be the commonly understood meaning, and when applied specifically to sex, it becomes *any intense desire or craving for sexual gratification and excitement.*

The problem, at least for Christians, is that we apply that meaning (because it's the only one we know) to the Bible passages that have Greek words that were translated into the English words "lust", "lusting", "lustfully", etc., and <u>the Bible words do *not* have that meaning</u>.

The Biblical Meaning of Lust

Matthew 5:27-28
"You have heard that it was said, 'Do not commit adultery.' But I tell you that anyone who looks at a woman lustfully has already committed adultery with her in his heart.

The Greek word translated into "lustfully" is epithumeo, and it means "to have a desire for something forbidden, to covet someone that belongs to someone else". Note that it does *not* mean "to imagine, to pretend, to fantasize".

But what does "covet" mean? It means wanting something or someone that belongs to someone else. Not wanting something *like* what someone else has, but wanting *the exact thing* that belongs to someone else.

Coveting is defined in Exodus 20:17, the tenth of the 10 commandments:

"You shall not covet your neighbor's house. You shall not covet your neighbor's wife, or his manservant or maidservant, his ox or donkey, or anything <u>that belongs to your neighbor</u>."

---

[12] Lust is a very serious issue because the sexually immoral will not go to heaven (see Holy Bible, Revelation, 21:8).
[13] http://en.wikipedia.org/wiki/Lust, as of August 1, 2008.

Think about that in non-sexual terms. Does this commandment mean that if your neighbor owns a car, then it's wrong for you to want a car? No, it means it's wrong for you to want your *neighbor's* car. You should not want *his specific car*, but it's fine to want to have a car in general. Otherwise, once one person in your neighborhood owned a car, no one else in the neighborhood would be allowed to want one!

Applying that principle to sexual desires, as it says, it's wrong to covet your neighbor's wife. That also applies to husbands from a lady's point of view. That means it's wrong to want your neighbor's husband in real-life. We hope it's obvious that if you're single, it does not mean that it's wrong to want some other man, a single man, to be your husband.

We can see this meaning of covet is a necessary part of the meaning of the word lust in Matthew 5:28. If "looks at a woman lustfully" meant merely thinking about sex with *any* woman, that would prohibit a husband from looking at his wife and thinking about sex, because he would be committing adultery in his heart. But a man can't commit adultery by having sex with his own wife, so Matthew 5:28 cannot apply to husbands looking at wives. The only way for Matthew 5:28 to be true, then, is for the term "lustfully" to include the meaning of coveting. Thus, it is committing adultery in a man's heart if he has a covetous desire when he looks at a woman who is married to another man.

Therefore, the Biblical meaning of "lust" is not equal to "thinking about sex", and it is not equal to "a desire for sex". In Matthew 5:28, **lust is a real-life desire to have sex with a person who is married to someone else.**

If you have a real-life desire to have sex with a married man, that means you really want it to happen. That's lust. If you see a good looking married man at Church and overhear that his wife is going out of town, and start planning how you can find an excuse to go over to his house, hoping he'll become so attracted to you that he won't be able to resist you, that isn't pretending, that's pursuing, and it's lust. If you really want a man's wife to die so that you can have the man, that's lust.

The word epithumeo also has a broader meaning than just its use in Matthew 5:28 which specifies an adulterous context. Remember the meaning includes the concept "to have a desire for something forbidden"? Epithumeo also appears in other passages such as Colossians 3:5, 1st Thessalonians 4:3-5, and 1st Peter 2:11.

These expand the definition to: **lust is a real-life desire to have prohibited sex**. So, if you have a real-life desire to have casual sex with a single man, or with an animal, those are also lust, since those are forbidden forms of sex.

What kinds of sex are forbidden? Every kind of sex with a person other than your spouse, and every kind of sex with animals.

Got it? Lust is *not* merely thinking about sex, and lust is *not* merely desiring sex.

There is another word in the New Testament, *aselgeia*, that is sometimes translated as "lust", but it's usually translated as *licentiousness* because that's a more accurate translation. That word refers to someone who is dominated by their sexual appetite, and give in to it with little or no restraint. Aselgeia is not a part of a normal sex drive, and is therefore not a topic for this book to cover in detail, because it doesn't affect the previous discussion comparing fantasy with lust.

Now let's look at 3 ways of thinking about sex...

Thinking About Sex

God established marriage, therefore he wants people to get married. God created us male and female and told us to fill the Earth, which means he wants us to have sex. God also gave us brains, so he wants us to think. And since our brains don't have an off-switch other than sleep, our minds have to think about something while we're having sex. There are 3 possibilities for sexual thoughts:

- **Lust**: real-life desire for prohibited sex
- **Mating**: real-life desire for sex with an acceptable person
- **Fantasy**: imaginary-only, unwelcome in real-life, unrestricted topics

Lust means you're thinking about a real-life desire to have sex with someone or something other than your spouse, and the Bible says clearly and repeatedly that this form of thinking about sex is sinful.

However, it's also possible to think about having sex with your spouse, or a potential spouse if you're single, and that is not lust, because even though it's a real-life desire, the object of your desire is an acceptable person. In the case of a sexual desire for a potential spouse, it's not lust as long as your real desire is based on getting married *before* fulfilling that desire.

That's a kind of legalistic explanation. The simple explanation is that thinking about sex is a normal, healthy, non-sinful part of marriage and of looking for a husband or wife. When looking for a spouse, sexual compatibility should not be the only consideration, but unless you're being subjected to an arranged marriage, it should be one part of the equation.

> **Thinking about sex is a normal, healthy, non-sinful part of marriage and of looking for a husband or wife.**

So, a real-life desire for acceptable sex is not lust. It's just part of normal married life, or before marriage as part of what motivates us in seeking a spouse. You see a good looking guy, you find out he's single, you pursue him or hope he pursues you, and you think about what it might be like to have sex with him. That's not lust, that's fantasizing to evaluate possibilities and consider if he might or might not be compatible enough to marry.

You can read more about compatibility issues in the Before Marriage chapter.

And that brings us to the third way to think about sex: fantasy.

Sexual Fantasy

In this book, we're using the word fantasy to mean the same thing as imagination[14], not a genre of literature.

Although the imagination is involved when we lust or have thoughts about sex with a spouse or potential spouse, real-life desire dominates the imagination in these cases.

Sexual fantasy, in contrast, is *imaginary-only*. Not only is it not dominated by real-life desire, it would be completely unwelcome in real-life. And that's what makes sexual fantasy different from lust:

Lust is real-life.
Fantasy is imaginary.

Remember that the Greek word epithumeo does *not* mean to fantasize. Fantasizing about sex is not lust, because it's not a real-life desire. Just because sexual fantasy often draws on the real world for ideas and imagery, that doesn't make it a desire for something real.

This difference is huge: one is actual, covetous desire, while the other is playful imagination. Let's emphasize this one more time this way:

Lust is real-life desire for forbidden sex, and sexual fantasy is a pretense that by definition is *not* real-life.

Imagination is part of who we are. It's part of how God designed us. While we're little children, we pretend our little stuffed bear is real, and we talk to it. A little older, and we're pretending that our dolls are having tea with us, or that our toy car is flying through the air. When we get a little older, we imagine what kind of job we might have someday, and we start imagining what married life might be like. While we're dating or going

---

[14] Imagination is a complex cognitive process of forming a mental scene that includes elements which are not, at the moment, being perceived by the senses. Despite being studied since at least Plato, well over 2000 years ago, it is not well understood by science. Nevertheless, "Researchers have found that imagery plays a significant role in emotion, motivation, sexual behavior, and many aspects of cognition, including learning, language acquisition, memory, problem-solving, and perception." – Gale Encyclopedia of Psychology

through courtship, we imagine what it would be like to be married to a particular person!

And imagination never stops, no matter how old we get! People imagine things all the time, sexually and otherwise, and imagination is part of a normal, healthy personality.

Okay, so far, so good, but there is another important characteristic of sexual fantasy we need to deal with: The unlimited range of creative concepts. In Biblically acceptable sexual fantasy, there are no restrictions on topics, issues, ideas, or even reality.

That last statement is based on the principle that sin is defined for us by the Bible, so if the Bible does not tell us something is sin, it is not sin. We know that having a real-life desire for sex with a person we are not married to is sin because the Bible tells us so. The Bible doesn't tell us whether or not brushing our teeth is okay, but we know it is because the Bible doesn't tell us it's wrong.

But doesn't the Bible have something to say about what kinds of things we should think about? Sure it does. Lots of things, in fact, and we think they're well summed up by Philippians 4:8: *"Finally brothers, whatever is true, whatever is noble, whatever is right, whatever is pure, whatever is lovely, whatever is admirable – if anything is excellent or praiseworthy – think about such things."*

At first glance, you might think this means that you should not think about wild sex fantasies, but if so, you need to look at it more closely. Encouragements like this either have to include mundane things, or be in addition to mundane things. We have to spend some time in our lives thinking about brushing our teeth, going to the grocery store, and many other mundane things. For example, unless you work full time as a pastor or missionary, you have to spend a lot of time thinking about the mundane tasks necessary to do your job. Come to think of it, even people with full-time spiritual jobs have a lot of mundane tasks to take care of.

So Philippians 4:8 isn't intended to prohibit certain thoughts, it's intended to encourage us to spend at least some time thinking about things that are loftier than mundane things. We should spend at least some time thinking about heroic role-model and uplifting types of things. So this passage, and others similar to it, tell us things that are good to think about, rather than things we are not allowed to think about.

That brings us back to the principle: sin is defined for us by the Bible, so if the Bible does not tell us something is sin, it is not sin. And if this principle is correct, and then there are no restrictions on sexual fantasies, because the only thoughts the Bible prohibits regarding sex are thoughts that are based on real-life desires for forbidden forms of sex, and it does not say anything about prohibiting imaginary thoughts of any kind.

Okay, but **how do you distinguish a real-life desire from a fantasy?** Suppose you lie in bed and dream about a particular married man being madly in love with you, and trying to seduce you. Is that a real-life desire or fantasy? You can tell by considering what your reaction would be if it happened in real life. If the married man were to appear in your bedroom and you wanted to have sex with him, then what you were thinking was a real-life desire, and lustful. However, if that married man were to suddenly appear in your bedroom and you'd scream and run, then what you were thinking was a fantasy. It's fantasy if you do not actually want him in real-life, and instead you just want to pretend.

Are you beginning to see it? If you imagine that a man breaks into your room and forces himself on you, you may enjoy that in your imagination, but *only* in your imagination, because if it happened in real life it would be an indescribably horrible thing.

Remember, the "lust" Jesus condemned is a real-life desire for forbidden sex, not a pretend-world fantasy.

James 1:14-15 describes real-life forbidden desires in general terms: *"...but each one is tempted when, by his own evil desire, he is dragged away and enticed. Then, after desire has conceived, it gives birth to sin; and sin, when it is full-grown, gives birth to death."*

When applied to the issue of sexual desire, this passage indicates that lust, if the person doesn't stop, will end up with the person taking real-life actions to fulfill their lust. Again, that's not fantasy, which specifically excludes real-life possibilities.

Think you understand the principles now? Then let's try the most extreme example...

What if you fantasize about wanting your neighbor's husband? Is that lust? It is not, not if it's truly fantasy, because *fantasy is not real-life*. As long as you don't actually want your neighbor's husband, you're *not* coveting *him*, you're only pretending something in which your imagination is based on the *idea* of him.

Based on the principles described above, then, in Biblically acceptable sexual fantasy, there are no restrictions on topics, issues, ideas, or even reality.

So, yes, you can fantasize about having sex with a real person, even if that person is married to someone else, because it's make-believe, a pretense. In fact, in your imagination, there can be three copies of your neighbor's husband! And they can all doing different things to you at the same time... in a space ship... while it's televised... while you kiss all three at one time because you have 3 mouths... *Because... it's not real!*

You can pretend that you're a kangaroo and another kangaroo is humping you, because that's *not real*, it's imagination. Or you're a kangaroo and you're having sex with a whale, or you're a tiny human having sex with a chipmunk, or you're a full-size human having sex with a giant chipmunk.

While having sex with a spouse, it's almost universal to mix real-life desire and fantasy, and your thoughts can jump all over the place many times in just a few minutes. And there's nothing wrong with it as long as *the real-life desire is always, only for your spouse.*

Suppose you and your husband get into bed naked and you want him and only him actually in your bed. But while he's playing with you or moving inside you, you pretend it's a man you know from work who's doing all that. Is that okay or not? Think of the principle of real-life desire: if you opened your eyes and saw your coworker on top of you would you be thrilled or terrified? If terrified, it means your real-life desire is truly for your husband, and your husband alone, so it's okay to pretend that he's *anyone*, or *anything*.

Hey, it's imaginary! Poof, that coworker you were pretending was on top of you is now the President, and poof, now it's someone you knew 20 years ago, poof, now you're the prom queen, poof, now all your office coworkers just turned into different kinds of bears and lions waiting to have a turn with you, and poof...

Wait a minute. How can you possibly have such wild sexual thoughts? How can you possibly think so many crazy sexual things while you're having sex with your husband? Because you're having sex *with your husband.*

Now it's time for one more principle. If you're a Christian with a real desire to be a godly person, the only way you can have wild fantasies like that while you're having sex with your husband, is by being secure in the *fact* that you are with your husband. **You know in reality that you are in your bed, with your husband, and *that* is what gives you freedom to imagine.**

Think of it this way. If you woke up with a man on top of you, what would your immediate thoughts be? One of two things will happen: Either you will assume it's your husband, or you won't be able to think about anything else except determining who it is. If you assume it's your husband and when you open your eyes or hear his voice to confirm it, you just continue having sex. If you assume it's your husband but then discover it's not, you realize you're being raped and you fight and scream. And if you wake up and you're not sure who's on top of you, you're going to fight to make the person stop until your brain can make sense of the situation and figure out who it is. Why will you react this way? Because in reality, you don't want to have sex with anyone other than your husband, and because you accept having sex with your husband as a normal, safe activity.

Did you catch the implication? *If you are not sure who you are having sex with, you <u>cannot</u> fantasize, because your entire body and all your thoughts will be in fight-or-flight mode.* It is *only* when you are safe and secure in the *certainty* that you are in your husband's *physical* arms that your imagination is free to soar.

What kinds of sexual fantasies do people have? Here are the results of a non-scientific survey Grandma Elizabeth conducted by phone and email with 35 wives and 34 husbands who had been married at least 10 years. The questions were based on fantasies during intercourse. Clearly, the women surveyed indicated more active imaginations during sex...

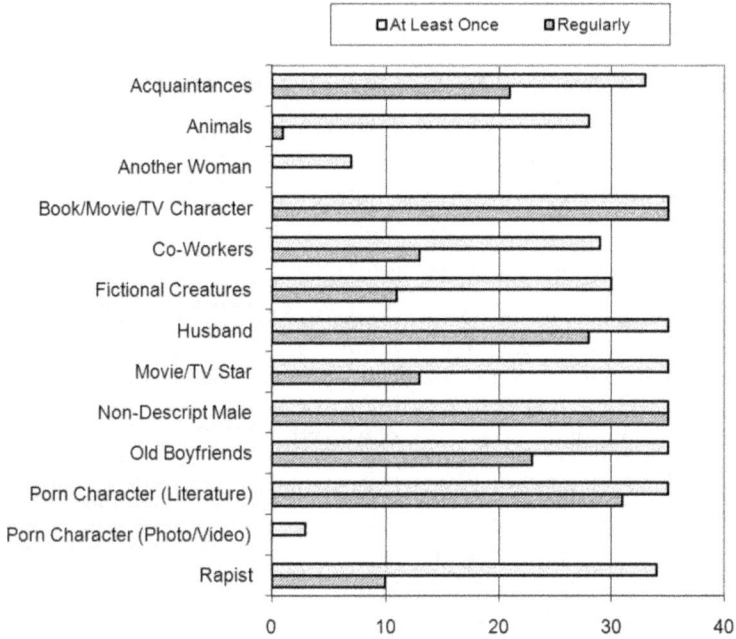

Figure 27. Female Fantasies

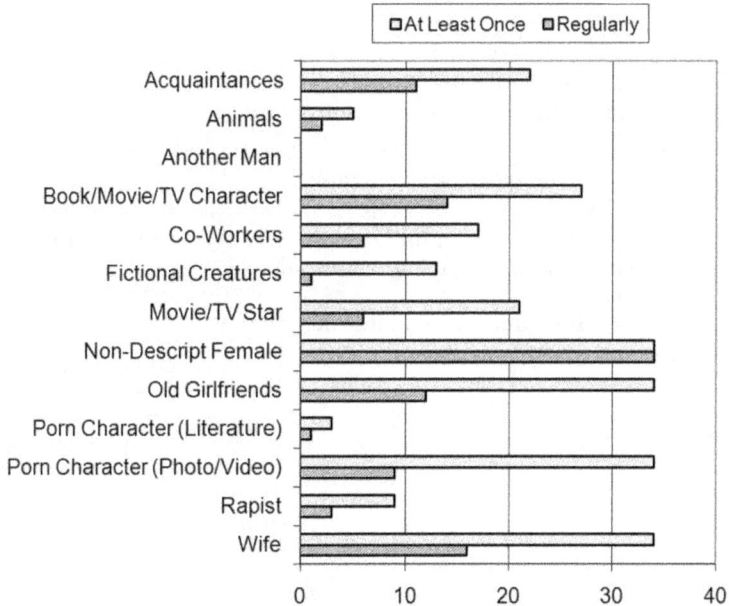

Figure 28. Male Fantasies

Fantasy In God's Design

God designed us with imaginations. He built imagination into us. And remember in Genesis 1:27 where it says he created us in his own image? He used His *imagination* to do that!

We use our imaginations from earliest infancy until we die, or at least until our brains quit working, and normal imagination for adults includes sexual fantasy. Put another way, normal people fantasize, and normal people who have sex fantasize about sex.

So, let's put that into a recap of everything we've covered in this chapter:

- Sex is normal.
- Fantasy is normal.
- Sexual fantasy is normal.
- Sexual fantasy is **not** lust!
- Lust is real-life.
- Fantasy is make-believe.
- Lust is a real-life desire for prohibited sex.
- Prohibited sex is sex with a person other than your spouse or with an animal.
- A real-life desire for sex with your spouse is not lust.
- Real-life thoughts of sex with a potential spouse is not lust if the desire is constrained by a stronger desire to wait until after marriage.
- In Biblically acceptable sexual fantasy, there are no restrictions on topics, issues, ideas, or even reality.

God gave us imagination, and it's okay to enjoy it, even during sex. Especially during sex!

PORNOGRAPHY

- What is Pornography?
- Growing Use And Acceptance
- Why Porn?
- The Bible on Pornography
- Advantages And Disadvantages
  - Negative Effects
  - Positive Effects
- Is Porn Okay?

Grandma's advice never talked about pornography before. Maybe that was because there wasn't any pornography available when Grandma's advice started being passed down. Now, it's extremely common, and sexual imagery has permeated society in the media, advertising, and conversation, so we decided we should include the topic from now on.

Grandma Elizabeth began researching, Grandma Dora and her husband began studying the Bible on related topics, Grandma Jennifer brushed up on relevant psychological topics, and those fueled numerous discussions among us. We can all say that we were surprised at some of what we learned.

We can say this right at the beginning: if both you and your husband avoid all pornography, that will work well. If either of you gets to the point where you need porn in order to become aroused, that's dysfunctional, and you should seek help.

What is Pornography?

Pornography, commonly referred to as *porn*, is sexually explicit media of any kind, including writing, pictures, videos, animation, video games, drawings, paintings, sculptures, audio recordings, etc. Hardcore porn specifically shows or describes aroused genitals or sexual intercourse and usually lacks significant story development. Soft-core porn, also known as *erotica*, ranges from seductively suggestive poses to full nudity and heavy petting. Pornographic writing is often referred to as *erotic literature* and is usually story-oriented.

The purpose of pornography is to stimulate the imagination of the reader, viewer, or listener, arouse them sexually, or facilitate reaching an orgasm. Material intended to be educational regarding sex is generally not considered pornographic, even if very explicit.

Pornographic photos and videos involve real-life sexual activity, while other forms of porn are based only on imagination. Reading, watching, or listening to porn, however, even real-life based porn, is all about fantasy for a normal person doing the reading, watching, or listening. Similar to reading a non-sexual novel or watching a movie, people tend to subconsciously imagine that they are involved in the story somehow, and making use of porn facilitates people creating their own sexual fantasies.

While it would be possible for creators of porn photos and videos to use only married couples, and thereby avoid actual fornication and adultery by actors, that rarely seems to be the case. First, there are many porn photos and videos of sex among more than 2 people at once, homosexual activity, and even bestiality. Second, based on testimonies of people who worked in this industry, even when the sexual activity is between one man and one woman, they are rarely married to each other in real life.

Also based on the testimonies of people who worked in this industry, it is common for some actors and actresses to experience severe guilt, shame, and depression, to regularly become intoxicated and engage in other self-destructive behavior. All this would be bad enough, but it is also very common for the women in these productions to be relentlessly exploited. While some women choose to get into porn knowing what it's like, others are drawn into it out of financial desperation or other hardships, and held there by fear, guilt, and shame. Others choose to work in porn because it often pays very well without requiring education, training, or serious job skills.

Growing Use And Acceptance

In the early 1900's, boys would eagerly take the Sears and Roebuck catalog to some private place and study the drawings of women wearing corsets, but that was about it for early American farming families.

Attitudes toward modesty and related issues seemed to become more liberal throughout the 1900's, as evidenced by swimsuits slowly evolving from full-bodied to string bikinis.

The first widely disseminated pornography in the United States began with Playboy magazine in 1953, followed rapidly by many competitors, and the very explicit novel "Lady Chatterley's Lover" republished in 1959. There was a great deal of resistance to their distribution in many communities, and by the U.S. Postal Service, but legal cases made it to the Supreme Court which ruled that the free speech clause of the first amendment to the U.S. Constitution allows for the creation and distribution of porn as long as it has some kind of content in addition to merely appealing to prurient interests.

Eventually, stores selling porn magazines were rarely picketed or busted by vice cops, and porn magazines in many subgenres became available in many stores. Simultaneously, a market was growing larger for "romance" novels, many of which contained sex scenes which became more and more explicit.

By the 2000's, pornography had proliferated in all forms on the Internet, and erotic literature continued to increase to new records. While pornographic photos, videos, and animations are primarily viewed by men, romance novels are read primarily by women.

In 1982 paperback romance novels reached $300 million in sales, and by 2004 it generated over $1.2 billion in sales. In 2005, romance became the most popular genre in modern literature, and a survey of readers found that they mirror the general population in age, education, marital, and socioeconomic status.

Why Porn?

A desire for sex prompts an interest in porn, and conversely, reading, viewing, or listening to porn prompts a desire for sex.

People who read, view, or listen to porn do so because they *want* to be sexually excited by it. It feeds people's imaginations, making it easier to fantasize about sex. Most people either fantasize as they read, view, or listen, or they store what they read, see, and hear in their memory to recall later. They may integrate porn-derived fantasies into their love-making while having sex with another person or use it to facilitate masturbation. Many men find masturbating to pornography easier and faster than having sexual intercourse with a woman.

The effectiveness of porn in helping men masturbate is the reason that fertility and sperm donation clinics stock their specimen collection rooms with magazines with pictures of nude women. With the pictures, it's easy and quick for a man to get to an orgasm. Without them, men take a long time or simply can't get to an orgasm.

Grandma Elizabeth spent some time studying the kinds of pornographic pictures and videos marketed to men, and decided to conduct an ethnographic experiment with her husband, "E". She and he sat in bed together as she showed him pictures and monitored his physical reactions, asking him to describe what he was thinking and feeling as he viewed each photo.

For the experiment, she put each photo into 1 of 24 categories of sexual conduct, ranging from a seductive-looking, fully dressed woman to group sex and everything in between. She also categorized the facial expression of the woman's face, if it was visible, along with the woman's age, body shape, hair color, and hair style, and she categorized the locations the photos were set in. The viewing time was varied from 1 second to 60 seconds. She also conducted the tests periodically over two months, and she showed some of the same pictures to her husband multiple times ranging from 15 minutes apart to over a month apart.

Want to know the results? Of course you do, but bear in mind that this experiment was limited to only one man, and that E, Elizabeth's husband, is a devout Protestant Christian. Here are Grandma Elizabeth's main findings, many of which surprised her.

- The only characteristic noted when E was repulsed by photos was that the woman appeared to be scared or in pain.
- The only characteristic noted when E was disinterested in photos was when the woman looked haughty, unhappy, angry, or disinterested.
- When E was repulsed or disinterested, he wanted to stop looking after only 2 or 3 seconds. In every other case, he preferred to vary his viewing time from 10-25 seconds. Based on discussions, this seemed to be so that

his imagination could create a story involving him in the scene.[15]

- In photos with a couple, in every case when E was not repulsed or disinterested, he imagined that he was the man. In photos of a woman alone, he imagined he was with her anyway. In photos that featured 2 men having sex with 1 woman, he imagined that he was both men simultaneously.
- In every case when E was not repulsed or disinterested, he imagined that the woman wanted to have sex with him, that she was aroused because she was thinking of him, or approaching orgasm because of how he was making her feel.
- The more enthusiastic the woman appeared, the quicker and more fully E became aroused.
- For the majority of photos, E imagined that the woman was his wife, and for the rest, he imagined that the woman was someone he had known in the past. In no case did E attest that he imagined that the woman was a contemporary acquaintance.
- In cases where a photo had 2 women and 1 man, he imagined that one woman was his wife and the other woman was a 2nd wife that he did not associate with anyone he had ever known.
- For each photo that E found arousing, he was highly aroused when viewing a particular photo for the first time.
- When being re-shown photos after the first time, only a very few were highly arousing every time. How stimulating the other repeats were depended on how long it had been since he had last seen them. Most photos were not arousing when reviewed within several days, whereas almost all photos that had originally been arousing were arousing again when reviewed after at least two weeks.

Grandma Elizabeth was initially surprised that E was not repulsed by photos that showed sex in semi-public settings, group sex, or mock bondage scenes. Upon questioning, it became clear that E was not picturing the scene as a real event, but as imaginary.

---

[15] E attested that had he been masturbating during the experiment, he would have preferred to look at some photos much longer while he played out a story in his imagination, based on the photo.

Grandma Elizabeth concluded that for her husband, the images fed his imagination only, and did not create or foster any lustful desires for E to have sex in reality with anyone other than herself.

We all found this study rather fascinating, and several other Grandma's and their husbands volunteering for a much more limited test. Grandma Elizabeth chose a set of 24 photos, and 5 other couples conducted one-time tests. Those results were mixed, with some husbands responding similarly to E, and others with widely divergent reactions.

In these tests, no sexual activities were presented that the wife disagreed with. For example, all 5 couples had already practiced anal intercourse before, therefore, the husband's viewing photos of anal intercourse prompted his imagination, but not a newfound desire to try anal intercourse. Were this experiment to be performed with a man who had never had anal intercourse, then it would have been more likely to result in stimulation of more than the imagination. If the husband viewing anal intercourse for the first time develops a desire to try it himself, the net effect may depend on his wife's response. If his wife agrees to have anal sex with her husband, his desires might be fully satisfied, as with the couples who participated in our experiment. If, however, a wife finds the idea so repulsive that she refuses to participate, it could result in the husband developing lustful desires to find a sex partner who would be willing to perform the kinds of sex his wife objected to. Grandma Yvette is certain that many of the married men who hired her as a prostitute (before she became a Christian) did so because their wives refused or were *reluctant* to participate in activities such as oral sex, anal intercourse, fantasy-based role-playing, gender-reversal, etc.

This is not to say that a husband's lust is his wife's fault if she refuses to participate in certain types of sexual acts, but to point out that it could be a factor. It seems certain that visual porn aimed at men and written porn aimed at women will both increase awareness of the many kinds of sexual activities possible. If a couple has previously been ignorant of some forms of sexual activity, pornography can increase awareness, *and increased awareness can create or expose incompatible desires.*

One of the goals of Grandma's sex advice is to make a soon-to-be bride aware of all forms of sexual activity so that she can decide before marriage what she is willing to try, and discuss it all with her groom before the wedding. If successful, it avoids a couple finding out after marriage that one spouse desires to experiment with all forms of sexuality within marriage while the other is too inhibited.

The Bible on Pornography

What does the Bible say about pornography? Nothing, directly. The closest issues in the Bible that we could find and may be related to the issue of pornography are exploitation, holiness, propriety, modesty, self-indulgence, and nudity.

Exploitation
Matthew 7:12 *"In everything, do to other what you would have them do to you, for this sums up the Law and the Prophets."*

We are to treat other people the way we want to be treated. At the least, this means we should not exploit anyone in order to create pornography, *nor should we spend money on porn that is based on exploitation and thereby finance it.* However, this particular point might not prohibit a person from creating pornography if no one is taken unfair advantage of in doing so, or from using free porn, or from using porn that does not involve living people. It could be a source of conflict between husband and wife if one approves using pornography while the other finds it offensive without exception.

Holiness
1st Peter 1:15-16 (Leviticus 11:44-45) *"But just as he who called you is holy, so be holy in all you do; for it is written: 'Be holy, because I am holy.'"*

When first considered, this passage might be considered as prohibiting the use of porn. However, this does not prohibit physical sex, nor does it prohibit sexual thoughts, as it is not possible to have consensual physical sex without some kind of sexual thoughts, nor is it possible to have an orgasm without having sexual thoughts. Since we are commanded in Genesis 1:28 to "increase in number" and "fill the Earth", that commandment indirectly requires us to have at least some sexual thoughts. Therefore, Grandma Synthia concludes, the meaning of the word "holy" does not exclude sexual thoughts, and as we explain in the previous chapter on fantasy vs. lust, we do not think it excludes sexual fantasies. If we are correct that a person can have sexual fantasies and still be holy, then it might be possible to read, view, or listen to some forms of porn and yet remain holy, despite that being a counter-intuitive idea.

We also think we should point out that if you think "holy" means you should not have any sexual thoughts at all other than the minimum required to create babies, then you should not watch any TV, movies, or read anything that might possibly prompt sexual thoughts. Even shows and books without explicit sex scenes may still prompt you to imagine sexual thoughts. And that would also seem to prevent you from reading the Song of Songs in the Bible, and all the other Bible passages dealing with sexuality, such as the incest of Lot and his daughters or the adulterous story of David and Bathsheba.

We think it should be clear that some sexual thoughts are not sinful, and if they are not sinful, they can be part of a Godly life. And that may mean that books, pictures, audio tapes, and other things that suggest or directly promote sexual thoughts, such as the Song of Songs, may also be compatible with a Godly life.

1st Thessalonians 5:22 *"Avoid every kind of evil."*

Well, this will definitely prohibit porn *if* porn is evil. And when we started out to form some advice regarding porn, we expected the Bible to clearly tell us that all porn is evil. But it didn't. That takes us back to the principle that if the Bible doesn't tell us something is evil, it's not evil. If some porn is evil because it exploits real people, that doesn't necessarily mean that other porn that doesn't exploit real people is also evil.

Propriety & Modesty
1Timothy 2:9 *"I also want women to dress modestly, with decency and propriety, not with braid hair or gold or pearls or expensive clothes, but with good deeds, appropriate for women who profess to worship God."*

1 Peter 3:3-4 *"Your beauty should not come from outward adornment, such as braided hair and the wearing of gold jewelry and fine clothes. Instead, it should be that of your inner self, the unfading beauty of a gentle and quiet spirit, which is of great worth in God's sight."*

Check it out, and you will discover that the admonition to dress modestly was specifically talking about not wearing rich, fancy clothes and accessories, and was not dealing with how much skin was exposed. Propriety means "with self-control or sobriety," but decency has the meaning of "bashfulness." Okay, bashfulness might apply to porn based on real-life people, but... honestly, this passage is talking about how Christian women should dress for Christian meetings. It doesn't apply to how a women should dress in the bedroom, obviously, and it really doesn't directly apply to the idea of movie actors portraying scenes, regardless of whether or not some of them occur in the bedroom during intimate encounters.

For our fellow Christians who think showing skin is bad in general, re-read 2nd Samuel, Chapter 6, where King David danced "with all his might" to celebrate the return of the Ark of the Covenant. One of his wives criticized him for showing too much skin, but it was apparently okay with God.

Self-Indulgence
Luke 8:14 *"The seed that fell among thorns stands for those who hear, but as they go on their way they are choked by life's worries, riches, and pleasures, and they do not mature."*

Okay, if sexual pleasure is the most important thing in your life, you've got a serious problem. However, bearing the context in mind, this passage is not saying that you should never be concerned about daily things, or that you should never have any money. Neither does it imply that you should never have any sexual pleasure. It just says that you should not let any of those things consume all your attention so that you can devote some time to spiritual issues.

Ecclesiastes 8:15 *"So I commend the enjoyment of life, because nothing is better for a man under the sun than to eat and drink and be glad. Then joy will accompany him in his work all the days of the life God has given him under the sun."*

This passage clearly states that it's okay to enjoy life. Neither of these passages directly address porn, but they do touch on the issue of self-indulgence. We put these here for your consideration, but we don't think this leads to a prohibition on using or creating porn.

Nudity
Okay, the Bible has lots to say about nudity! Well, actually it has the words arowm in Hebrew and gymnos and gymnotēs in Greek, which are usually translated as naked or nakedness, and it simply means a person is not wearing clothes. And it does not

say that nakedness is sinful or even sinful under certain circumstances.

Mostly it refers to nakedness as a condition of dire poverty, and encourages us to provide clothes to those who need them, or it sites nakedness as a reason for shame. Adam & Eve were naked and not ashamed, until after they sinned. Then they became ashamed of their nakedness and started wearing clothes.

However, even if nakedness always produces shame, that doesn't make it evil. Evidence that it's not evil comes from Isaiah 20:2-3, where God has the faithful prophet walk around naked for 3 years. This is a good example of why we should not make assumptions about what is good and evil, but depend on the Bible to instruct us.

Advantages And Disadvantages

Some proponents won't admit that there are negative aspects of porn, and some opponents won't admit that there are positive aspects. Almost everything in life has both advantages and disadvantages, and we want to be as honest as possible in covering this issue. Here are some negative effects that we identified:

Negative Effects

1. Produces a downward spiral.
2. Severe danger to immature people.
3. Promotes objectification of women.
4. Exposes incompatible sexual desires.
5. Can result in feelings of betrayal.
6. Can result in unrealistic expectations.
7. Can result in exploitation.
8. Can lead to dangerous sex.
9. Can result in guilt and shame.
10. Can promote immoderate masturbation.

Downward Spiral

Curiosity drives people to explore porn with every kind of sexual activity, and though this can apply to women, it's more common with men viewing pictures and videos. Porn in every form is easily available on the Internet, in many cases for free. They

may begin by looking at nude women, but with a few more
mouse clicks they can see unrestrained hardcore porn of orgies,
bondage, bestiality, and rape, and curiosity compels them to
explore it all.

Danger to Immature Minds

All pornography is dangerous to all children, all young teens,
and everyone else who has not yet formed a mature perspective
on sexuality. The danger is due to their inability to fit sexual
practices into a complete, healthy view of life, due to their
limited knowledge and their inability to distinguish normal from
abnormal behavior. People with an undeveloped framework for
understanding sexuality cannot distinguish behaviors of a well-
adjusted married couple from dangerous, make-believe
behavior of people being paid to perform titillating acts.

When children or those with insufficiently developed minds
read or see pornography, the mental images can become
building blocks in their mental and emotional development.
Common results are that a vulnerable person may come to think
of sex as dominating all other forms of male-female interactions,
that sex dominates all life activities, that aberrant sexual
behavior is normal, or that sex is nothing more than instinctual.

How prevalent is this problem? **The Justice Department
estimates that 90% of children aged 8-16 have been
exposed to pornography on the Internet.** A software
security company found that 47 percent of school-aged children
receive pornographic spam daily, and representatives from the
pornography industry told the Congress' COPA Commission[16]
that as much as 20-30% of traffic to some pornographic Web
sites are children.

Blocking children from reading, seeing, or hearing porn will
help the children, but that won't protect adults with vulnerable
adults. The impact on maladjusted adults is hard to measure,
but it can be severe, as indicated by the testimonies of serial
killers such as Ted Bundy, Jeffrey Dahmer, and Gary Bishop.

Objectification

Young men being exposed to pornography may be the primary
reason many develop a perspective that women are little more
than sexual objects that exist primarily or exclusively to satisfy
men's sexual desires.

---

[16] www.copacommission.org

Incompatible Desires

Couples can be married their entire adults lives with very limited sexual practices and be perfectly happy. However, a spouse's desires can change, and the result of the differences can range from beneficial, to insignificant, to catastrophic. Sometimes pornography can trigger such changes.

On the bad side, a couple can be married for years with very limited sexual practices and be getting along okay, when the man starts looking at visual pornography and develops a desire to try anal sex which his wife opposes. Or a wife may read pornographic stories and decide she wants more sexual adventure that the husband has no interest in.

Incompatible sexual desires may also appear without porn playing a role, but regardless of how it arises, how a couple works on such incompatible desires might result in a stronger relationship or it can result in a destroyed marriage.

In "An Affair of the Mind",[17] the Christian author wrote about her husband starting to use soft-core porn, then visiting strip clubs, then hiring prostitutes. We Grandmas don't doubt her heartbreaking story. However, in contrast, most of our husbands have significant experience with pornography, and it has not lead to any sexual activities outside our marriages.

The author of that book also points out that infidelity in the mind is linked to infidelity in the body, and Grandma absolutely agrees with that – that's the definition of lust! But in our previous chapter, we present evidence that fantasy is not the same thing as lust. But can porn lead to lust? Grandma Synthia believes that lust may certainly lead a man or woman to porn, but that for a man or woman with a faithful heart, porn will not lead them into lust.

Feelings of Betrayal

This seems to usually be an issue with women feeling betrayed by men viewing pornographic pictures or videos, and not men feeling betrayed by their wives reading pornographic literature.

Grandma Jennifer, a psychologist who has counseled many women regarding sexual issues, notes that it has been common among those patients to think written porn is okay for them, but that their husband viewing visual porn is an act of betrayal.

---

[17] *An Affair of the Mind*, by Laurie Hall, Tyndale House, 1998

Grandma Jennifer tries to show them that it's two sides of the same coin, with varying degrees of success.

A common complaint seems to be, "I should be enough for my husband," yet these same women will reluctantly admit that their own minds "wander" before, during, and after sex, meaning that yes, they do fantasize about having sex with other men.

Grandma Synthia believes that the truth is that both husbands and women require fantasies, and it is the nature of fantasizing to be unconstrained. Women tend to feed their fantasies with language-based porn and men tend to feed their fantasies with visual-based porn. A husband or wife with a faithful heart who seeks fantasy is not betraying their spouse. A husband or wife with lust in their heart is unfaithful in their minds, and is likely to betray their spouse regardless of the use of pornography.

Unrealistic Expectations

Immature people using porn often develop expectations based on what they read, hear, or see to set a mental standard for sexuality and sexual partners, instead of merely using it as a tool of fantasy. Such standards are not realistic, and may lead a married person to think their spouse is an inadequate, inferior sex partner. That kind of distortion can prompt lust, and a woman may seek a man to have an affair with, or a married man may seek prostitutes who dress and act more like the women in porn films. When the new sexual partners don't measure up to the unrealistic standard, the person with that immature standard is likely to continue to seek new partners, and never find satisfaction.

Exploitation

There have been numerous testimonies by women who participated in real-life pornography productions who felt compelled to act against their desires or against their wills by fear of violence or fear of becoming destitute. That is especially evil since there seems to be no shortage of women eager to participate for the money or fame.

Dangerous Sex

Companies that create real-life pornography usually have a lot of different actors having sex with each other and often forego condoms, resulting in the spread of sexually transmitted diseases.

Guilt and Shame

Both producing and using pornography can result in guilt and shame. Many Christians consider themselves addicted to porn if they recognize they have a long-term desire for it, especially those who believe that using pornography is sinful.

Immoderate Masturbation

Pornographic literature, videos, and all the rest can be so stimulating that it sometimes prompts users to masturbate alone, even if they have a spouse and that spouse is available and willing to have sex. This is especially true if the person using porn is hiding their use from their spouse. The most significant negative characteristic of porn and masturbation is when the use of porn promotes masturbation to the point where it reduces a person's interest in their spouse.

Positive Effects

Some proponents won't admit that there are negative aspects of porn, and some opponents won't admit that there are positive aspects. Almost everything in life has both advantages and disadvantages, and we want to be as honest as possible in covering this issue. Here are some positive effects that we identified:

1. Porn in any medium can teach a person new methods of sexual activity.
2. Porn facilitates sexual fantasies.

Educational Value

Pornography describes or shows a wide variety of sexual activity. That's one reason some people don't like it. It is obvious, though, that if you read or watch something you've never seen or read about before, you learn about it. Yes, you can have sex education material that is not intended to arouse the reader or viewer, and that's fine. But it is also possible to learn new techniques from sex material that is intended to arouse.

There are some women who have no objections to written porn who strongly object to visual porn. Here's what one of our Grandma's had to say about the benefit of a wife studying the visual porn that is so popular with men:

Grandma Heather: If you think video pornography shouldn't be watched by godly women, consider this: video pornography wouldn't exist if the people who create it didn't earn profits from it, they wouldn't earn profits from it if men didn't pay for it, and men wouldn't pay for it if they didn't find it more appealing than anything else they could do with their spare money. That's basic economics. And that means <u>video pornography is an accurate reflection of what men find sexually stimulating</u>. I decided when I got married that I wanted to be the best I possibly could at getting my husband aroused and getting him to climax, and I decided to study male-oriented porn in order to learn as much as possible. I believe it has helped me be a better wife than I otherwise might have been.

Sexual Fantasy

No, women don't like their men looking at porn of other women. But for many men, looking at female nudes or at sex videos, it's the same for them as it is for women who read porn – it's a prompt to stir their imagination, and nothing more. For them, it's a fantasy trigger, not something that creates or even reflects a desire for someone else.

Is Porn Okay?

Based on everything discussed above, including the issue of fantasy vs. lust in the previous chapter, Grandma Synthia concludes the following about the acceptability of pornography:

1. All pornography is *extremely* dangerous to vulnerable minds. That includes all children, all young teens, and everyone else who has not yet formed a mature perspective on sexuality. Sexually active does not mean sexually mature. In modern American culture, many teens become sexually active long before they acquire a mature perspective on sexuality.
2. Creating or using imagination-based porn is okay for adults with a mature sexual perspective.
3. Creating porn based on real-life is okay for adults with a mature sexual perspective *only if* the live participants are not exploited, do not engage in dangerous sex, and sex only occurs between husbands and wives.

4. Using pornography based on real-life images or video is okay for people with mature sexual perspectives if they do not have a spouse who feels betrayed, and if they do not finance exploitive porn (by purchasing it or paying fees).

Why don't we just say real-life based porn is wrong? Honestly, it seems a little unfair to say that the written form of porn is okay but photos and videos aren't, because it's primarily women who prefer the written form and men who prefer the visual form. And, for men who use visual porn only to stir their imaginations, it's effect is no different than the written form is for women.

It seems to us that using imagination-based porn and milder forms of real-life-based porn is similar to using alcohol: it is too dangerous for some people to use at all, but for mature adults, it's okay to use in moderation. This conclusion is dependent on the principle that sexual fantasy is not the same as lust, which is the primary topic of the previous chapter.

MASTURBATION

Masturbation is when you touch your own genitals, or make something else touch them, in order to stimulate yourself sexually, usually to the point of orgasm.[18] If you've ever masturbated, or if you masturbate frequently, you're not alone.

---

[18] Some people use the term "masturbation" to refer to one person using their hands to massage another person's genitals, but in this book we refer to that as *manual* sex.

The Reality Of Masturbation[19]

After studying the Bible, science, and sexual research, and conducting formal and informal studies of our own, Grandma Synthia has come to believe the following, which we'll cover in more detail through this chapter and in related material that appears elsewhere in this book:

- Masturbation is a normal part of sex for most people.
- Masturbation is not sinful.
- Fantasy is a normal part of masturbation.
- Fantasy is **not** lust.
- Fantasy is not sinful.
- Most people who masturbate do it a lot.
- Most people hide their masturbation.
- Women tend to masturbate a lot less while married, and men tend to masturbate a little less while married.
- Christian men and women usually feel guilty about it because they think it's wrong, and try to resist the desire, but frequently fail.
- Masturbation is part of God's design.
- Masturbation can be a part of a Godly life.
- Masturbation can improve marriages.

We are sexual creatures. We are *more* than sexual creatures, but we are *also* sexual creatures.

With healthy bodies, starting with puberty, hormones create sexual desires within us, very much like how we get hunger pangs when we go for long enough without eating.

Many Christians, and many people influenced by Christianity, have been in a long-term state of denial regarding masturbation as a normal, acceptable form of sexual relief, primarily due to confusing lust, which is forbidden, and fantasy, which is normal and not forbidden. See the earlier chapter, Fantasy vs. Lust.

---

[19] WebMD has a summary article on masturbation titled "Your Guide to Masturbation, and it's available at http://www.webmd.com/sex-relationships/guide/masturbation-guide.

Who Masturbates?

Most people masturbate, including Christians. Most men masturbate a lot, including married men.

The percentage of Christians who masturbate, and the frequency of masturbating by Christians appears to be only slightly less than the general public, despite the fact that there is near universal condemnation by Christian pastors and counselors.

Various studies indicate that at least 80% of men, and perhaps as much as 95% of men, masturbate regularly, and that includes married men.

Most women who masturbate while they're single stop it when they get married and have regular sexual intercourse, but most men do not. For most men, regular sex with their spouse only decreases the frequency of their masturbation.

Men who masturbate usually do so most frequently when they are in their teens and twenties, with most masturbating daily, and declining in frequency as they get older. Few couples have sex as often as daily. If you do, then the odds are fairly good that your husband may not be masturbating at all. But many men masturbate *more* than once a day, so even if you have sex with your husband daily, it's no guarantee he's not still masturbating sometimes.

Repression of masturbation is still strong in some groups, including with many Christian pastors and counselors, but that doesn't seem to reduce the practice.

Grandma Dora provides a relevant story from her husband "D":

> *Grandma Dora: D began masturbating as a teenager about once every day or two. As a Christian, it bothered him greatly, and it made him feel very guilty. He didn't want to, he wasn't reading porn, and he would frequently repent and ask God for strength to do better. But nothing changed.*
> *This pattern continued until he entered a seminary to study to become a pastor. He lived in a dormitory with 8-9 other young Christian men also studying to become pastors.*
> *In the dorm, D usually got up before anyone else, and his morning routine included taking a shower in the*

dorm bathroom. He frequently relieved his sexual urges there through masturbation, and then did his best to ignore the issue until the next morning.

Each of the men in the dorm were assigned various chores in rotation for one month at a time. After awhile, D was assigned the task of cleaning the bathroom.

While cleaning the shower, he discovered the drain stopped up with hair that was heavily choked with semen. This made him very upset, as it had never dawned on him that the fact that the shower never drained well was because of his masturbation. His mind ran wild wondering how many of the other young men might suspect that he was masturbating in the shower, and thought about how humiliated he would be if it became widely known.

He cleaned the drain thoroughly, and determined to either stop masturbating, or if he couldn't, he would at least make sure he cleaned up after himself.

The next morning while in the shower, he noticed that the shower immediately filled with standing water, as it always had. He examined the drain, and it was once again clogged with some hair and lots of semen. Obviously, at least one of the other young men had masturbated in the shower. This happened every day. D decided that he had had enough. He reported the situation to the Dean, who called an emergency meeting of all the residents of the dorm to discuss sexual thoughts and masturbation. Much to D's surprise, every young man confessed to the "sin" of masturbation, and there was a long period of prayer for each of them to be "delivered" from bondage to that sin.

Finally! This would set him free!

D successfully abstained from masturbation the next morning, and apparently everyone else had, as the shower drained without hindrance. That night, however, D had a wet dream. And the morning after that, the drain was stopped up again, by more semen than he had ever had to clean out at one time before. And he also could not refrain from masturbating.

D concluded that he would have this problem until he got married so he could properly satisfy his sex drive with his wife. That was when we met, and we married after a short courtship. However, marriage did not stop D from masturbating, it only reduced how often he did it. Unknown to me for a long time,

*since I was only in the mood for sex once every few
days, D was relieving himself almost every day in
between.
Year later, D confessed this to me, and we simply
made it part of our lives together.*

D and the other young men in his dorm were about as serious as
anyone could be about not masturbating in order to live Godly
lives. If anyone could overcome it, they should have been able
to. The fact that they were not able to is strong evidence that it is
not something that needs to be overcome in order to live Godly
lives.

Despite the fact that most people do masturbate, most people
don't talk about it. American society has become very tolerant of
the idea, but not of discussing it. The fact is, people hide their
masturbation. Why? Here are some possibilities:

Why do people hide the fact that they masturbate?

- If married, because they're afraid their spouse will
  disapprove of their masturbation, or even worse, that
  they will disapprove of *them*.
- Because it is intensely personal and private.
- Because they think it is sinful.
- Because they think it might be sinful.
- Because they think other people might think it's sinful.
- Because society considers it a taboo topic, and a "bad"
  thing, regardless of religious opinions.

Repressing Masturbation

Some 3rd world cultures promote masturbation, while others go
to extremes to prevent it. Social discouragement is one thing,
but some backward, ignorant, foolish Islamic cultures practice
the surgical removal of the clitoris of girls, supposedly to
prevent women from masturbating, to reduce the likelihood that
they will commit adultery, and to reduce the likelihood they will
have sinful sexual thoughts.

This maiming, known as *Female Genital Mutilation (FGM)*, is
condemned by most Moslems, but not enough is being done to
stop this barbaric practice, which impugns the reputation of
Islam as well as damaging or destroying the lives of many
thousands of women. FGM is often performed without
anesthesia or sterile instruments.

Part of the sales from Grandma's Sex Handbook will be used to fight this practice and to support surgery that helps the victims of FGM.

Is Masturbation Okay?

Is it okay for a Christian to masturbate? Does God condemn it, or discourage it?

Suppose your husband's libido is much stronger than yours, and he needs orgasms far more frequently than you do. You may be willing to have sex with him as often as he wants. But what happens when his employer requires him to travel to another city for a few days? Sure, you can ask him to forego any orgasms until he gets home. But that means he may be going to business meetings "fully loaded". That doesn't mean he'll be looking for an excuse to have an affair or hire a prostitute, but it does mean that his body will be telling him, frequently and possibly loudly, that it wants relief. But while there are some men who find it very easy to ignore their body's cravings, but there are others for whom it is very hard. However, if it's okay for him to masturbate, he can go to his hotel room in private, unload in a few minutes, and in his business meeting tomorrow his body won't be interrupting all the time. Why send him to the grocery store hungry, if you get my drift?

Well, maybe you think masturbation's wrong, but you decide to compromise and you won't do it, but you'll agree to your husband masturbating... sometimes, under specific circumstances, with prior approval.

Well, that's a compromise, all right, but that doesn't make it a good one. Is masturbating a sin, or not? If it's a sin, are you suggesting that you'll approve of your husband committing it and risk having his soul condemned to hell for eternity? That's not a very nice compromise for him. On the flip-side, it's not a sin, then it's okay, for your husband and for you.

What does the Bible say about masturbation? There is exactly *one* passage that *might* refer to masturbation. Genesis 38:9-10 contains these snippets: "...he spilled his seed on the ground... What he did was wicked in the Lord's sight, so he put him to death also." Okay, that sounds like it *might* be masturbation, and God definitely does not like whatever it is. But that's the problem with taking snippets out of context. Read the full passage from verse 6 through verse 10, and it's clear that what the guy did wrong was intentionally avoid getting his dead brother's widow pregnant.

If you study the cultural rules of that time, you learn that the firstborn son in a family got a double share of inheritance. Women got no inheritance, and depended on their sons to take care of them in old age. And if one son leaves a widow and no son, any remaining brother is obligated to father children with the widowed sister-in-law until she bears a son.

In this case, Judah had three sons. The oldest married Tamar, but died before she bore him any sons, so she's got no retirement plan. The second brother, Onan, is now obligated to father children with her until she has a son. But if Tamar bears a son by Onan, it is he who will get the double share of inheritance, and there will be a 3-person split. If Tamar never bears a son, Onan will get the double share, and there's only a 2-person split. That means Onan gets 25% of his father's estate if he fathers a son for Tamar, but he'll get 66% if he does not father a son for her. So, Onan was greedy and did one of two things: he either had intercourse with Tamar but pulled out just as he began ejaculating, or he just did the whole thing with his hand. Either way, Tamar wasn't going to get pregnant that way, and she could expect to be destitute, and possibly starve to death someday.

So, the thing that Onan did that was wicked wasn't that he might have masturbated, but that he failed to live up to his responsibility to his sister-in-law and he did it out of greed. Got it? We can't be sure from that passage that Onan did masturbate, but even if he did, that wasn't the wicked thing.

Despite there being a lot in the Bible that talks about sex and sexual relationships, nowhere else in the Bible is there anything that talks about stimulating yourself to the point of orgasm.

Let's look at the Big Rules of the Bible, the 10 Commandments, the 3 Commandments, and the 2 Commandments:

The 10 Commandments (Exodus 20:1-17)[20]
1. Only God.
2. No idols.
3. Honor God's name.
4. Respect the Sabbath.
5. Honor your Mom and Dad.

---

[20] Grandma Anne's Unauthorized Version (GAUV)

6. Don't murder.
7. Be loyal to your spouse.
8. Don't steal.
9. Don't lie.
10. Don't covet.

The 3 Commandments (Micah 6:8)
He has showed you, O man, what is good. And what does the Lord require of you? To act justly and to love mercy and to walk humbly with your God.

The 2 Commandments (Matthew 22:37-40)
Jesus replied: "'Love the Lord your God with all your heart and with all your soul and with all your mind.' This is the first and greatest commandment. And the second is like it: 'Love your neighbor as yourself.' All the Law and the Prophets hang on these two commandments."

Okay, number 7 of the 10 covers adultery. None of these directly address masturbation. Nothing else in the Bible does either. Grandma's conclusion is: **The Bible does not say that masturbation is wrong or sinful.**

Recent History Of Christian Perspectives On Masturbation

100 years ago, the "learned experts" in the medical field diagnosed many women with a variety of complaints as having the disorder of *female hysteria*, and would treat it in their office with water sprays or industrial-sized vibrators applied primarily to their clitorises until they induced a mysterious *hysterical paroxysm* that relieved all their symptoms... for a few days. A *hysterical paroxysm* is now called *orgasm*.

As recently as 50 years ago, many in the medical field and most parents prejudiced by medical practitioners, were still warning their sons that masturbating was self-abuse, sinful behavior, and that it would cause – take your pick – insanity, blindness, weakness, epilepsy, or baldness.

The "sexual revolution" of the 1960's made huge changes in American society, and reduced many sexual inhibitions. For example, oral sex is thought to have been fairly rare before that, and became quite common afterward due to the willingness of many people to experiment more sexually.

Well, Grandma's clan has been enjoying masturbation, oral sex, and sexual experimentation between husbands and wives since at least the mid 1800s, because we didn't derive our beliefs from doctors or society, but from the Bible, reasoning, and traditions over multiple generations. And the fact that many of our ancestors lived on farms may have also been a factor.

According to Grandma Flora, when you grow up tending livestock, and your family's prosperity depends on animals having sex to create baby animals, animal sex was common knowledge, and breeding techniques were frequently discussed. Without the hum of air-conditioners, children hearing sex noises from their parents' bedrooms was unavoidable, and it was no secret to youngsters that people created babies the same way the livestock did. And it wasn't a big deal.

In 1976, Zondervan first published *The Act of Marriage* by Tim and Beverly LaHaye, and it was the most sexually explicit Christian advice book until now. The LaHaye's were widely respected as Christian leaders, and the book was a run-away best seller. It is still in print, and has a lot of great information, but it is from their perspective alone. Though Grandma Anne can recommend it for additional reading, don't take everything in it as Gospel. In particular, Grandma Synthia strongly disagrees with what they concluded regarding masturbation.

The LaHaye's said that masturbation was an unacceptable practice for Christians for 7 reasons, and we're now going to rebut them one-by-one.

1. Fantasizing and lustful thinking are usually involved, and the Bible clearly condemns such thoughts. (Matthew 5:28) No, it condemns lust, which is *not* the same thing as fantasy, and we've devoted an entire chapter to debunking this fallacy. See Fantasy vs. Lust.
2. Christians who approve of masturbation do so only because their reasoning has been corrupted by Humanists. That's an ad hominem fallacy. It doesn't matter if a conclusion is compatible with a Humanist perspective, it only matters if it's right or wrong.
3. Masturbation frustrates God's design of two people of the opposite sex being dependent on one another. No, it doesn't. High percentages of people have always masturbated, and the world population has soared anyway. Those billions of babies didn't come out of test tubes... couples have intercourse *in addition to*

masturbation. (And even if it were to reduce population growth, with 6 billion people on the planet, we've pretty well satisfied the requirement to increase in number.[21])

4. <u>Guilty feelings result from masturbation.</u> Well, there's a self-fulfilling prophecy. They tell Christians it's wrong, Christians can't stop themselves from doing it anyway, and feel guilty because the LaHaye's and others say it's wrong. A little later, we'll address the fact that consciences can be useful guides, but they can also be *wrong*, so they should be considered, but should not control decisions alone.

5. <u>Masturbation by single people will remove a reason to get married.</u> Hello? How many parents have begged their children not to get married because they're too young, but the kids insist anyway because... they want to have sex! If there were any doubts in the past, they should be gone now: Masturbation by single people helps them to be able to delay marriage and having children. *Delay*, not *avoid*.

6. <u>Masturbation is a "cop-out" when a husband and wife have sexual or other conflicts that make intercourse difficult.</u> Grandma says it's wrong if a person masturbates in order to withhold sex from their spouse, or if they masturbate so often they eliminate their desire for sex with their spouse. Grandma also says that's very unlikely to happen, as most married spouses who masturbate do it because their spouse doesn't want to have sex. Most would prefer to have sex with their spouse if they were able and willing.

7. <u>Masturbation defrauds a wife, and she will feel unloved and insecure.</u> Grandma says a wife is not defrauded by masturbation if she gets as many orgasms as she wants, despite additional masturbation by her husband, and her husband's masturbation will only make her feel unloved and insecure if she doesn't understand it. So read this chapter and you will understand masturbation, and you can feel completely loved and secure regardless of whether your husband masturbates in addition to having sex with you.

Okay, we hope you now understand that masturbation can be okay, both before and within marriage. But what about those feelings of guilt?

---

[21] Holy Bible, Genesis 1:22

Objections of Conscience

If you think something is wrong and you do it anyway, you'll feel guilty. That's a good thing. However, it is possible to believe something is okay, do it, and still be bothered by your conscience.

Although 1st John 3:19-20 is talking about having compassion and helping other people, there is a logical implication in it that relates to this issue. *"This then is how we know we belong to the truth, and how we set our hearts at rest in His presence whenever our hearts condemn us."* This shows that it is possible for our heart, our conscience, to be wrong. That doesn't mean that we shouldn't pay attention to our conscience, it just means that our conscience is not a perfect judge.

Sexual reservations run deep for most Christians, and even if you conclude from the Bible and by reasoning from the Bible[22] that masturbation is not a sin, it may still bother your conscience and make it difficult for you to do. This is a case where you may be able to *train* your conscience.

Yes, you can control your conscience, at least to some degree. If you know something is sin and you do it anyway, eventually your conscience will stop bothering you. 1st Timothy 4:2 refers to this as a "seared" conscience. Well, the opposite is also true, even if it's more difficult. If you know something is *not* sin and you do it anyway, eventually your conscience will... well, bother you less. It may not quit bothering you altogether, but it will at least bother you less.

Holiness And Masturbation

Can you be holy if you practice masturbation?
Well, can you be holy and have sex with your spouse? We hope that's an obvious "yes". Can you be holy and have an orgasm? We hope that's also an obvious "yes" since God's the one who designed our bodies that way.

And here, Grandma Dora has a very surprising sex tip. Well, maybe you won't be surprised, but all of us other grandmas were. And **this may be the best sex tip in the whole book.**

> ***Grandma Dora:*** *Shortly after I got married, I started wondering what God thought about while my husband "D" and I were having sex. My Grandma*

---

[22] Isaiah 1:18

*Flora told me a lot about sex before I got married, but
she didn't talk about that. And it really bothered me.
"D" was in seminary, having devoted his life to God,
and I wanted to be a Godly wife. But how could God
not see what we were doing, since He sees
everything?*

*I started studying everything I could find in the Bible
that talked about sex, and I didn't find my answer
there. Then I began trying to pray about it, and God
reminded me of many other passages that don't talk
specifically about sex, but that deal with all of life,[23]
which includes sex, and His all-encompassing love for
us. And there I got my answers.*

*God loves us, and gives us good gifts, and sex is a gift.
And, we are to give thanks for His gifts!*

Give thanks for sex? Yes!

*I began to give silent thanks to God when my husband
and I would start kissing in bed! I gave thanks as I
felt my dear husband moving inside me! And then one
time, I even gave thanks when a wave of orgasm
came over me! I cried out, 'Oh, God, thank you!', and
it was not in vain, but in praise!*

*That orgasm set my husband off and it was the first
time we came at the same time! We laid there and I
cried. After assuring my precious husband that I was
crying for joy, I continued to give thanks. And I've
been giving thanks ever since.*

*Years later, "D" asked me to try rubbing my clitoris
while he moved in and out, so that we could try to
have an orgasm at the same time again. I had never
masturbated before, because even though my
Grandma Flora had said it was okay, I wasn't
convinced. For my husband's sake, I made a very
reluctant attempt, but I got no pleasure from it, I was
embarrassed by it, and I quit. I could tell "D" was
disappointed, and that bothered me.*

*I continued to think about it, study the Bible about it,
and pray about it. I found nothing in the Bible to
indicate it was wrong, but I just didn't want to. For
me... I didn't want to masturbate just so I could have
a few fleeting seconds of having a good feeling. But I
did want to please my husband, and I couldn't forget
how disappointed he was, not that I hadn't had an*

---

[23] As one of many examples, my favorite verse of that time is the most
surprising verse in the Bible: Zephaniah 3:17 "He will take great delight in you,
He will quiet you with His love, He will rejoice over you with singing!"

orgasm, but that I hadn't been willing to do this thing for him, with him.

Well, it was my habit in those days to read a chapter from the Bible each morning, in order, and I had just finished the book of Revelation and it was time to start over, beginning with Genesis, chapter 1. I didn't stop there though. I kept going to the end of chapter 2: "The man and his wife were both naked, and they felt no shame." No shame… together, naked, and no shame. I prayed right then and I made a decision: I was going to do my level best to fulfill my husband's once-asked but never fulfilled request.

That night, after putting the children to bed, I put three towels down on the bed, one on top of the other, in the center, and took all my clothes off. "D" knew I meant to have sex, but he asked why I put down three towels. I said it was to make sure the oil didn't soak through. Then I brought out a small bottle of baby oil, and I told him I had a surprise. I waited until he got busy in a missionary position then asked him to change to a sitting position while I kept lying face up. He was happy to comply, and he watched intently as I took the baby oil and poured a small amount on my clitoris. He was surprised.

I put the bottle down and told him I was really going to try. I could tell he was about to ask "try what," but he didn't need to ask when I put my hand down there and started rubbing.

My! Never mind how it made me feel, my husband was shocked, and then aroused like never before. And probably louder than ever before. And he shook the bed as never before, finishing almost immediately before falling over onto me.

I expected the children to wake up and ask what all the noise was, but they slept through it. "D" told me how much that meant to him, as I thought about how little I had actually done, and how it had been rather pleasant, and… just possibly, a little shorter than I would have preferred. A few minutes later, however, I learned the night was not over.

"D" asked if he could do it again, and I said okay, of course.

This time he didn't finish right away, and I had as long as I wanted to experiment. And we talked, "D" and I, and he moved in and out, and I rubbed myself, and I actually enjoyed the rubbing, but that wasn't the best part. The best part was my husband knowing

*I had done this for him, and the appreciation he spoke
and showed in his eyes.
At least, that was the best part for awhile, and for
keepsake memories, but after awhile, I started
behaving differently... I started breathing rapidly,
and a minute later I couldn't keep from moaning and
writhing. Then I looked up for a moment and "D" was
watching, almost glowing with happiness, and I could
handle no more. I thought I would break the bed. I
don't know how long it went on, but it was wave after
wave, and somewhere in there I felt "D" having
another orgasm, and then I was so loud I thought I
must have woken the children.
Well, there never was a knock on the door asking
what was wrong, but there was another
repercussion:
I had never been able to bring myself to tell my
husband what felt good to me and what didn't, except
when something hurt, but that changed, much to "D"'s
delight!
Ever since that wonderful night, I've been able to tell
him when he does something that I like, I've enjoyed
sex more, and I've even been able to ask him to do
particular things to me.
And ever since, I've been giving thanks to God for sex
in general and orgasms in particular. I even heard
"D" use one of our code-words for sex in a public
prayer of thanksgiving!
I would have been too embarrassed to tell my story if
we hadn't made this book anonymous, but I hope my
testimony will help you live your life with all the joy
God intends for you – including while God is enjoying
watching you have an orgasm!*

Here's another example regarding holiness and marriage:
Suppose a husband becomes a quadriplegic, permanently
incapable of having sex in any way, so he can't help his wife have
an orgasm. Well, why does a husband want his wife to have an
orgasm? Because it makes him feel like he's doing his duty? Or
because he desires for his wife to experience the pleasure? If
he's a loving husband, he desires for her to have orgasms for her
sake, not for his sake. That won't change when he becomes an
invalid. Here are two options for a couple to handle this
situation.

The conventional way is apparently that the wife won't have any
more orgasms while he is alive, or, if she masturbates, it's done

in secret. Either way, as far as the husband knows, his wife is no longer having orgasms. How does that make him feel about his failure to help his wife experience pleasure? Not good.

An alternative scenario is for the wife to get alone with her husband, climb into bed with him, and tell him how much she loves him, and how she remembers all the wonderful times he was inside her, all the wonderful times he used his tongue to stroke her clitoris. And as she tells him these things, she strokes herself manually, building to an orgasm, in bed, beside her husband, and as she climaxes, she calls out his name. Then as the orgasm subsides, she strokes his face and tells him what a wonderful man he is, and how she will treasure their intimate times for the rest of her life. Now how do you think he will feel? Relieved and giving thanks to God that his wife has enjoyed sexual pleasure despite his disabilities? Well, if he thinks she shouldn't have an orgasm without him physically causing it, this would make him disappointed or angry, but if his interest is in her well-being, he'll be thrilled.

Are you surprised that Grandma Synthia thinks that the ideal scenario is for a husband and wife to agree that masturbation is part of God's design, and that they should integrate masturbation into their sexual repertoire?

1st Corinthians says: "It's better to marry than to burn." As in burn with sexual desire. Why? Because if you're burning with sexual desire, you're far more vulnerable to sexual temptations. Rushing into marriage is better than remaining sexually vulnerable. Well, masturbation does not remove the option of getting married, but it can reduce that pre-marital vulnerability, and thereby helps avoid rushing into marriage.

Advantages of Masturbation

People usually discover masturbation as ignorant teenagers, and immediately learn that it feels better than anything else they've ever experienced, it causes no apparent harm, and it helps them relieve their sexual tension. They may also discover that it can relieve depression, stress, and lead to a higher sense of self-worth.

Masturbation can be very valuable in relationships where one spouse wants more sex than the other, which is most relationships, as it provides a balancing effect and thus a better overall relationship. This can be especially important when couples are separated by business trips or long military deployments.

Mutual masturbation, when a husband and wife stimulate themselves in the presence of each other, allows a couple to reveal physically what makes them feel good, rather than trying to describe it verbally. Witnessing your spouse masturbate is an educational opportunity to find out the methods that please them, helping you learn some of the ways your husband or wife enjoys being touched.

For those who would otherwise engage in casual sex, masturbation provides a method of sexual relief without the risk of disease and pregnancy that comes from sexual promiscuity.

Sexual climax, from masturbation or otherwise, usually leaves a person in a relaxed and contented state. This is frequently followed closely by drowsiness and sleep, especially when someone masturbates in bed, so masturbation can help overcome insomnia when a spouse is not available, willing, or interested.

Like sexual intercourse, masturbation also raises the heart rate, and thereby acts as a cardiovascular exercise, and can help lower blood pressure.

With little downside, it's no wonder so many people do it regularly.

Female Masturbation

If you touch your own genitals in a manner intended to produce pleasure and result in an orgasm, you will:

A. Not shock God, who designed your body to have sexual pleasure, including orgasms.
B. Not disappoint God, who gave you a clitoris whose only function is to produce pleasure.
C. Learn more of what your body is capable of, so you'll know what your husband can help you accomplish.
D. Learn more about which things increase your sexual response and how, so you can help your husband learn how to give you more pleasure.

E. Gain more control over your sexual responses so that you can sometimes try to have an orgasm at the same time as your husband.

God designed your body, so you can't surprise Him with it, and you can't disappoint Him by using a gift He gave you in a way it was designed to be used.

Female Masturbation Techniques

Women usually need a romantic fantasy and physical stimulation of the breasts and clitoris. The clitoris is especially important, because it has more nerve endings than any other part of your body. In fact, for some women, the clitoris is often too sensitive to simulate directly. In those cases, massaging around the clitoris is done instead. Inserting an object into the vagina is also very common.

Here are some itemized suggestions:

Toyless Stimulation:
- Set up a soothing environment.
- Do it in a hot shower.
- Do it in a warm, soapy bath.
- Massage your breasts.
- Use your fingers to massage your clitoris. Lick your fingers for lubrication.
- Insert one or more fingers into your vagina.
- Insert a well-lubricated fingertip into your anus.
- If you have large enough breasts (or if your breasts sag enough!), you can suck on your own nipples.
- Use thigh-squeezing. Rotate your thighs inward to apply pressure to the clitoral area, release and repeat.
- Use erotic literature to stimulate your imagination.
- Use erotic pictures, movies, or audio to stimulate your imagination.
- Ask your husband to strip-dance for you.
- Ask your husband to penetrate you while you masturbate at the same time.
- Do it in an ever-so-slightly risky location such as at the office after hours, in an office toilet stall, or at night in your car in a location where you can't be seen (try in your garage, if you have one!).

Toy-based Stimulation:

- Use ben-wa balls in your vagina and while they're inserted, flex your legs, walk, dance around, or use a rocking chair. These are small, hollow balls that each contain a small weight that rolls around inside, and require muscle control to keep them in.
- Use a vibrator to stimulate your clitoris. All of them can be controlled by hand, and a few can be worn in a harness.
- Use a dildo or vibrating dildo to stimulate your vagina in general, or your A, G, or U-spots in particular.
- Use a rabbit vibrator to stimulate your vagina and clitoris simultaneously. A "rabbit" gets its name from the clitoral section on the first models, which used a pair of rabbit-ear shaped extensions to cup the sides of the clitoral hood, rather than massaging the clitoris itself.
- Use a triple action rabbit to stimulate your vagina, clitoris, and anus at the same time.
- Use a pulsating jet of water from a flexible shower hose
- Use a stream of water from a tub faucet or Jacuzzi.
- Use a string of anal beads to stimulate your anus both on insertion and on removal.
- Use gentle nipple-clamps.

Larger and harder-to-hide toys include:

- Use a Sybian saddle-mounted vibrator which combines a rotating dildo and clitoral stimulator.
- Use a "fucking machine" which uses a motor to thrust a dildo back and forth.
- Use a "fucking chair" which thrusts a dildo up and down as you rock in the chair.

How To Reach Orgasm

A small percentage of women have great difficulty in reaching an orgasmic climax. There are many reasons why that might be the case, including physical problems that may require the intervention of a doctor. Another might include guilt, and we hope this book will help alleviate that. But others may have difficulty due to fear, anxiety, or doubt. If you're married, these issues may be magnified when having sex with your spouse. If that's the case, we offer this guide to try to help you achieve orgasm through masturbation so you can become accustomed to it, and eventually have orgasms with your husband.

If you aren't convinced that masturbation is okay, then don't do it. If, however, you're convinced that it's okay, then you can try to learn to have an orgasm, all by yourself. If you decide to try, remember you don't have to have an orgasm the first time, or the first few times. That's okay, and you also don't have to have an orgasm every time.

To accomplish your goal, you'll have to touch yourself or make something else touch you. For the first time, start slow, and you can go as slow as you want, and quit as soon as you want. You can always try again later.

Remember, this is just a guide, and you can do things as differently as you wish.

Although you can do this anywhere that you can be in private, you can choose a place where you can set a romantic atmosphere if you want to. A classic is in a bathroom lit only by candles, in a bath of warm water with bath oils and bubbles, with soft orchestral music in the background. With bath oils, you may not need any other lubrication.

Don't just launch right in, but use some relaxation techniques first. Lean back, and take a deep breath and let it out slowly. Relax all your muscles starting with your neck. Tense each muscle tightly, slowly release the tension until it's all gone, then move down to another muscle and repeat until you get to your toes, and then scrunch and release them, too. Take another deep breath and let it slowly out.

Move a hand to each breast and slowly slide your hands back and forth just an inch or so, savoring the sensations. Then move each hand to the base of a breast and squeeze very gently as you move your hands toward the nipples. Try to experiment a little by using a firmer squeeze or going all the way to the nipples. Move your hands so that a fingertip can touch each nipple, and gently squeeze each breast and hold as you lightly touch the nipple and caress it with the fingertip.

When you're ready for more, draw your knees up and press your hands firmly against your skin as you slide your hands down the outside of your torso, hips, thighs, and shins, as you concentrate on the feeling where your hands are touching. Switch to a light touch and bring them back up the same places. Focus on the sensations as you keep the light touch and go down over the same path again, switch to a very firm press of your fingertips as you lower your legs, dragging your hands back up again.

When you're ready for more, begin repeating the breast touching, then move one hand to your pubic hair while you continue to stroke your breast and nipple with the other hand. Weave your fingers through your pubic hair, then press your fingertips down and drag them upward a few inches. Separate your legs some and flatten your palm and push your hand down until your fingers can reach your clitoris and labia. Lightly explore your clitoris and labia with your fingertips, sensing their shape, softness, and texture. Use your fingers to slowly separate your labia and any matted hair so that you can stroke up and down all the way from your clitoris to your anus. Put all your fingers over your labia and squeeze your legs together as you notice the sensations on your clitoris, labia, and thighs. Keep squeezing your thighs together lightly and move your hand up and down ever so slightly as you concentrate on the feelings it creates.

When you're ready for more, slowly begin to stroke your clitoris. When stroking the clitoris, experiment with different amounts of pressure from medium to very light. If your clitoris is too sensitive to stroke at all, reach a little higher and stroke the clitoral hood, or massage the area just above the clitoral hood, and again experiment with different amounts of pressure. Try massaging the area on either side of the clitoris and note how that feels differently from the clitoris and clitoral hood.

When you're ready to try to reach an orgasm, the easiest way for most women is to stroke the clitoris or around the clitoris with a very steady rhythm, while massaging one or both breasts with your other hand. Take deep breathes and release them slowly. Feel your body responding, and allow yourself to move freely as a sensation build throughout your body. Continue to massage yourself and breathe deeply, accepting the buildup of feelings, and when you're ready, allow it to overflow.

When you've had an orgasm or want to stop trying for now, squeeze your thighs together and release. Relax your hands and arms, and take a deep breath, releasing it slowly. Take another deep breath as you silently give thanks for a body that was designed to experience physical pleasure. Breathe normally and enjoy the peace and stillness.

Male Masturbation

If your husband is like many men, he'll hide the fact that he masturbates, and may initially deny it if asked about it. Most men hide their masturbation, including from their wives, and getting your husband to masturbate in front of you or with you may require more trust on his part than anything else ever will. Why should you acknowledge or share in your husband's masturbation? Because **accepting your husband's masturbation is part of accepting *all of him* and *who he is.***

Unless there's something wrong with your husband, he probably started masturbating long before he met you, and he will continue to do so when he gets horny and you aren't available. Or you may be available but he won't want to impose or interrupt you. And that may be far more often than you might think.

Why do married men still masturbate? It's usually fast, easy, he doesn't have to wait until you're present or willing, and he doesn't have to feel like he's imposing on you when you just had sex recently. These reasons apply to all married men.

In addition, the "easy" aspect is critical for men with physical or health limitations, especially any of the many problems that can make their muscles weak or painful: it takes little effort to move a hand up and down while masturbating, compared to the vigorous whole-body exercise usually used to have sex with you. If you truly have your husband's best interests at heart in such circumstances, you should encourage him and help him relieve his sex drive in the easiest way possible.

In addition to making it clear to him that you approve of him masturbating, you can participate in his masturbation by stripping for him, sexily dancing naked in front of him, or... masturbating yourself in front of him. Providing such erotic visual stimulation can help your husband's imagination get him to an orgasm much faster, and for a man with muscle weakness or pain, that can be a huge gift to him to help him quiet his sex drive's demands. If you aren't available or able to provide such visual cues, you should consider allowing him to view some forms of porn for the purpose of getting past the plateau stage to orgasm.

How A Man Masturbates

The physical aspect of male masturbation is almost always done by using a hand around the penis, stroking up and down, and often lubricated with saliva, pre-ejaculation fluid, soap, oil, or personal lubricant.

The other hand is sometimes used to stroke or caress the scrotum, the perineum, the anus, or the P-spot. Applying firm pressure on the perineum just before ejaculation can heighten the intensity of orgasm. The P-spot must be reached by inserting a finger into the rectum and pushing lightly on the front wall (toward the penis).

The mental aspect of masturbation for a man, as with a man reaching orgasm through intercourse, seems to require erotic images, either from memories or from observation during masturbation. There's a reason that sperm donation clinics stock their specimen collection rooms with magazines with pictures of nude women. With the pictures, it's easy and quick. Without them, men take a long time or simply can't get to an orgasm. And no orgasm, no sperm donation.

Grandma Elizabeth conducted an experiment where she picked porn pictures for her husband to look so she could study his reactions (see the Pornography chapter). In addition to the direct results of the experiment, she discovered that the effort significantly increased the level of trust and intimacy between herself and her husband. In fact, it was so successful in that regard, that she continued to collect pornographic photos for him. She chooses primarily pictures that have only a woman or one man and one woman, and the woman always has a big, happy smile, if her face can be seen. She occasionally has sex with her husband in a position where he can view the pictures while they have sex, and she makes him welcome to view the pictures when he masturbates without her.

Elizabeth's story was inspiring enough that several of us other Grandmas have tried it with notable results in the areas of intimacy and trust, even though we and our husbands were already comfortable with masturbating in front of each other. We all started out believing that our husbands would use the images to foster their own imaginations, and not real-world lusts, and after many discussions with them, we remain convinced that it has not lead them into uncontrollable sexual desires and depravity.

Male Masturbation Toys

Most men masturbate without using sex toys, but there are several that can be used. These include:

- **Cock Rings**, these tightly encircle the shaft of the penis or the penis and scrotum, and help to maintain an erection in the case of erectile dysfunction, or to delay orgasm.
- **Cock Ring Vibrators**, these small vibrators attach to cock rings and provide pulsing sensations.
- **Butt Plugs**, these are inserted into the anus, either repeatedly or inserted and left in while the anal sphincter muscles are contracted and released.
- **Butt Plug Vibrators**, these are small vibrators built into butt plugs and provide pulsing sensations to the nerves in and around the anus.
- **Prostate (P-spot) Vibrators**, these vibrators have slender necks and a bulb on the end, and the bulb is gently pressed against the prostate gland through the wall of the rectum.
- **Artificial Vaginas**, more commonly known as *pocket pussies*, are cylinders filled with a material that feels flesh-like and has a narrow opening in the center. A man slides this up and down his penis.

Hot Sex Tip:

The single sexiest thing a man or woman can do is...

Smile.

GREAT SEX

Any man and woman can have sex. But it takes knowledge and effort for a man and woman to have *great* sex. Here's how Grandma groups her great-sex tips:

- Beyond Basic Sex
- Honeymoon Sex
- Devoted Sex
  - Husband-Building
  - Relationship-Building
  - Mastering the Quickie
  - Deep-Throating
  - Comfort Sex
  - Sensuality Improvement Guide
- Pregnant Sex
- Sex After Children
- Senior Sex
- Alternative Sex
- Problems Affecting Sex

Beyond Basic Sex

What's the difference between ordinary sex and great sex?

Ordinary sex is no more than the minimum to make a baby, and may leave both husband and wife unfulfilled physically or emotionally. Ordinary sex is not much different than animals satisfying their sex drive when the female is in-heat.

Great sex means both the husband and wife pay attention to all of their spouse's sexual needs, and that means constantly improving your ability to satisfy your spouse's sex drive, building your spouse's ego, increasing intimacy, increasing trust, and... better orgasms. More orgasms, longer orgasms, more powerful orgasms, and more endearing orgasms. Orgasms are a key to enjoying sex and keeping your husband satisfied, which are the goals of this book.

And great sex means great foreplay! Lots of flirting and teasing each other, showing body language that says "I want to have sex with you", or occasionally seducing your spouse. Anything and everything that shows your desire, anticipation, and appreciation.

For wives in particular, *providing* great sex means they must *enjoy* great sex! Husbands don't just want wives that are *willing* to have sex, they want wives who *want* to have sex with them. And good husbands want to give their wives orgasms, so wives have to learn how to enjoy sex enough to have orgasms, and build enough intimacy and trust with their husbands to be able to help the guys learn how to help their wives get to an orgasm.

Many young wives assume that simply being willing to have sex as often as their husband wants is fulfilling their sexual duty to them, but to many men, nothing makes them feel as complete as being able to give their wife an orgasm.

Your husband needs to know that he is fulfilling his sexual duty to you, and that means you have to enjoy sex, and you have to let him regularly bring you to orgasm.

Married women tend to be very conservative and inhibited regarding sex, while prostitutes tend to be very liberal and uninhibited. Can you guess any reasons why some husbands might be tempted to use prostitutes? You're right if you think that sex with an uninhibited, active prostitute is more exciting for a husband than having intercourse with a wife that's totally passive. But if you're sexually assertive, and fully explore and enjoy your sexuality with your husband, it won't make you dirty or sinful, it will make you *considerate*... and fulfilled.

Honeymoon Sex

Some of Grandma's granddaughters will have sex before marriage, and others will have read all about sex, but this part is for those who have abstained or not read much about it. You can also become divorced or widowed and have subsequent honeymoons, but this topic is for the first-timers. Nevertheless, much of it may apply to second marriages, since every man has different sexual desires and abilities.

You're young, you get married, and you have a honeymoon. In America, many newlyweds seem to think that a honeymoon is basically a short vacation to have lots of sex and start getting used to living with each other, such as learning to sleep in bed with another person. While that may be true, **your honeymoon is also the best time to develop an**

openness with each other than can last your entire lives together. We'll get back to this issue, but first things first...

Your wedding night is the first night of your honeymoon and of your married life together. If you're a virgin, your wedding night is the first time you have sex, and your hymen may still be intact.

The hymen is a thin layer of membranous tissue that partially closes the opening to the vagina. Some societies have relied on examining the hymen at the time of marriage to confirm that a woman is a virgin, but that isn't reliable, because it is thin enough that it often becomes torn by physical activity, especially in athletes.

The main act of sex is putting your husband's hardened penis into your vagina. When that happens, if your hymen is intact, the penis will usually tear it a little bit, and there will be a small amount of bleeding, about like when you lost a baby tooth, or just a little bit more. Some women have said it didn't hurt at all, but others have said it hurt quite a bit.

Grandma Sylvia thinks **the level of pain a young woman feels when her hymen is broken often depends on the state of her sexual arousal.** If a bride is not aroused and is highly anxious, her muscles may be very tense and she may focus on the discomfort. However, if a bride is highly aroused sexually, it is much more likely that the breaking of her hymen will be a minor sensation that is quickly forgotten.

Once your husband's penis is inside you for the first time, he's going to move it in and out until he has an orgasm. You may also move around, but he definitely will. When he has his orgasm, his penis will squirt some semen into your vagina, and when he pulls out, the semen will start leaking out of you, and it will be a little sticky at first. **If you don't want a small mess on whatever you're laying on, be prepared with a towel or something to clean up.** Your hubby will also need a cloth to wipe his penis off. His semen will total a tablespoon or two of liquid, and your vaginal juices will add a little to that.

Another thing that you can expect: **sex can be noisy!** When a man or woman gets to the point of orgasm, it's often accompanied by involuntary moaning, groaning, or even roaring. That's not the only kind of noise, however. When sex is vigorous, a bed can be very noisy from stresses on bed springs and the joints in the bed frame. And if the headboard is close to the wall, vigorous thrusting can cause the headboard to hammer against the wall. And there's still more: When sex is vigorous and wet from sweat or vaginal lubrication, there can be all kinds of loud schlopping and flopping noises from two human bodies interacting with each other.

How can you keep the noise to a minimum? Based on many years of experience by many Grandmas, our advice is: Turn on a fan or stereo for background noise, pull the bed a few inches away from the wall so the headboard doesn't hit the wall, and forget everything else. Everything else may sound loud to you, but that's because you're right there where the noise is being made. It's not as loud outside your room, if it can be heard at all. If you're really bothered by noise from the bed, try having sex on the floor or standing up. Best of all, just don't worry about it! You're on your honeymoon and you're having sex – that's what people do on honeymoons! Enjoy it all as you experiment with different positions and techniques and learn the various noises that come from each!

If you're on your period on your wedding night, you have several options. You can lay on top of an adult disposable diaper to catch the blood while in the missionary position, you can have sex in the shower, or you can skip vaginal intercourse until your blood flow slows down or stops. You and your new husband should agree on this decision. If you're one of the women who hates the idea of having intercourse while on your period, you may need to put aside your concerns for your husband's sake. If he's been anxiously awaiting this moment for weeks or months, it might be extremely frustrating to him to ask him to wait.

Now back to the issue that your honeymoon is the best time to develop a lasting openness with your husband. **Take advantage of your honeymoon** and the fact that your new husband and you are just beginning to learn to live together. **Your expectations are now at their most flexible, so make a point of exploring your sexuality with each other.** Build intimacy and trust by taking turns examining each other's genitals in detail, by telling each other about sexual fantasies you've had, and by beginning to get comfortable with showing your spouse what makes you feel good.

It's especially important for you to teach your husband how to help you reach orgasm. Few women can achieve an orgasm from vaginal intercourse alone, but most women can reach orgasm if their husband will lick their clitoris long enough (cunnilingus).

A few women can't reach orgasm without the high-speeds of a mechanical vibrator applied to their clitoris. Some women can't reach orgasms at all, and if this applies to you, you should see a physician to determine if you have a physical problem, and if not, see a psychologist to see if you have an emotional problem.

Note that unlike most porn videos, a man and woman achieving simultaneous orgasms is actually rare, and many couples never do. In marriages with inconsiderate husbands, the couple frequently have vaginal intercourse and the husband has an orgasm, while the wife does without one. There's no excuse for this, and the best solution is usually for a considerate husband to lick his wife's clitoris until she reaches orgasm, and then have intercourse until he does. Getting his wife to orgasm this way is highly arousing to most husbands, and most women love to be penetrated immediately after reaching orgasm through oral sex. So, **try the "ladies first" approach, and see if it works as well for you and your husband as it does for most couples.**

If your husband has intercourse long enough without an orgasm, his penis may begin to soften before he wants it to. The easiest, fastest way to get him re-inflated is to put him in your mouth for a few minutes (fellatio). You can move your mouth up and down on him, move your tongue around while he's inside your mouth, or switch back and forth. If he doesn't have a medical problem, that usually works very well. Note that many medications make erections more difficult, and if that's the case, he might want to ask his doctor for Viagra or something similar.

If you want the most intimate relationship possible, you need to become comfortable masturbating in front of each other. You don't have to masturbate to the point of orgasm, but that's okay, too. But just initiating masturbation in front of your spouse requires far more trust than sexual intercourse does. It may take you a long time to reach that level of trust, but your honeymoon is a great time to get started.

In fact, the hump-rub is a favorite of many of the Grandma's in our family, and with their hubbies. A hump-rub is when the husband is thrusting in and out of the wife's vagina while she rubs her own clitoris. A deck-chair or spooning position works well for this, but any position will work that lets the wife get a finger or vibrator to her clitoris. If you really want to try to have a simultaneous orgasm, the hump-rub is the best method to try. And, even if it's not quite simultaneous, it's still a lot of fun!

Devoted Sex

"Devoted" sex covers the period of time after your honeymoon and before your first pregnancy.

When you're young, which is when most honeymoons occur, sex-related hormones can dominate your libido and your mental processes. Orgasms are also easier to come by when you're on a vacation specifically for having sex. If you get too tired, you just lounge around a little while, then when you're not too tired anymore, so you can go at it again.

After the honeymoon, you may want to have sex just as much, but you'll have less time for it due to work, school, or other demands.

> *Grandma Jennifer: When "J" and I got married, J was working a 12-hour night shift, and I was working 8-5 during the day and taking evening classes. On the weekdays we saw each other in passing each morning, and were often too tired for sex, but we made up for a lot on the weekends!*

Despite any difficulties, you need to keep your sex drives satisfied. Toward that end, in this section we'll discuss these sexual issues: relationship-building, husband-building, quickies, comfort sex, and a sensuality improvement guide.

Relationship-Building

There are many issues that can be part of building a strong relationship between a husband and wife, such as finances, communication, physical and emotional security, conflict resolution, and of course, sex. This book only deals with sexual aspects of building a marriage relationship.

Making a continual effort to improve your sex life can help you and your mate develop common interests and pastimes, become more trusting, and become more intimate.

How do you build trust and become more intimate using sex? By trying new things together. Not every time you have sex, but at least once in awhile. It can vary from something simple, such as trying a new position, to something more difficult. Bear in mind, though, that what is more difficult for some people may be easy for others.

What is the most intimate trust-building sex you can have with your husband? Mutual masturbation.[24]

You think sexual intercourse is intimate? That pales in comparison to masturbating in front of your spouse, and your spouse masturbating in front of you. Nothing is more intimate, nothing requires more trust, nothing makes a person feel more vulnerable than that. If and when you and your husband can reach this point, you will have earned your doctoral degrees in intimacy, because **sharing masturbation is the most intimate thing you and your husband can do**.

Some couples may be able to do this on their honeymoon, while others may take years to get to this level of trust, and others may never reach it. Your honeymoon is the ideal time to try it, if you both agree, because the idea of a honeymoon has set your expectations for new sexual experiences.

Why masturbate with your spouse when you can have intercourse? The best reason is simply because it builds trust. In addition, it proves to your spouse as nothing else can that on occasions when you don't feel like having sex, you approve of him relieving himself.

Some women go their whole lives without ever masturbating, and are quite content with their sex lives. Most women masturbate from around puberty until they get married, and then they stop masturbating or rarely masturbate. Some women continue to masturbate regularly after marriage, in addition to having sex with their husbands.

In contrast, almost all men masturbate. A lot. Including husbands. That's right, even most married men masturbate. *A lot*. What most husbands do not do, most of the time, is tell their wives.

Even though most husbands won't tell their wives that they masturbate, Grandma Yvonne tells us that most of the men who use prostitutes are very uninhibited and don't mind masturbating in front of a hired girl. (Although that usually only happens during foreplay, such as while the women are undressing, stripping, lap dancing, etc., since the men are

---

[24] "Mutual masturbation" means the husband and wife each masturbating simultaneously in front of each other. In this book, we use the term "manual sex" to refer to using your hands to stimulate your spouse.

paying for more than just watching.) She believes that **many men who use prostitutes are much less inhibited with hired girls than with their own wives**. Why? Because they know the hired girls won't reject them, or they won't look down on them when they lower their guard and play with themselves. Or perhaps because they don't care what a hired girl thinks about them. But if a man is afraid his wife will think less of him if he reveals his true inclinations, that is extremely strong incentive to hide those inclinations from you. And that is the opposite of relationship-building.

The truth is that it is very likely that your husband will masturbate while married to you, and it is likely that he will do it a lot. A big factor (but not the only one) is that most husbands need sexual relief far more often than most wives. For many married men, masturbation is often just a way to quickly and easily satisfy an inescapable hunger. By masturbating, they avoid being sexually frustrated and reduce the possibility of being sexually tempted at work or any other occasions away from home.

Repeating from the chapter on Masturbation, why should you acknowledge or share in your husband's masturbation? Because if he's part of the huge majority who masturbate even while married, accepting **your husband's masturbation is part of accepting *all of him* and *who he is*.**

You can *accept* your husband's masturbation as a normal mechanism for him to relieve his sexual urges. And you can *tell* your husband you accept it. Or you can *prove* to him that you accept it. How can you prove it? By coaxing him into doing it in front of you, *for* you, and *with* you.

Masturbating "for you" means that as he masturbates in front of you, he is not only relieving himself, he is entertaining you.

Masturbating "with you" means you have to masturbate yourself at the same time he's masturbating. Even women who masturbate while married may find it very difficult to do so in front of their husband. You may have the same apprehension of rejection as your husband. If, however, you can overcome your fears, you'll discover it has an extremely powerful effect on your husband. **For a husband, watching his wife masturbate may be the most erotic thing he will ever see.** The fact that you are doing it despite fear of rejection, that fact that you are doing it to please him, will make an indelible impression in his mind, and help make your marriage bond incredibly strong.

How hard will it be for you and your husband to be able to masturbate together? That depends on how strong your sex drives are, how often each of you would masturbate alone (if at all), how much you trust your spouse, and how much your spouse trusts you. The only way to find out for sure, is to talk about it, and then *try it*!

Hot Sex Tip: Try sucking one of your husband's nipples while he sucks one of yours!

Husband-Building

Building a *relationship* is about a living connection between you and your husband. Building your *husband* is about helping him become all God intends him to be. A wonderful way that you can help build your husband is by being the best sexual partner you possibly can.

You will always be a powerful influence on your husband, and your sexual relationship is a big part of that.

- Every time you have sex, you remind him that you desire him.
- Every time you give him an orgasm, you remind him that you care about his needs.
- Every time you allow him to give you an orgasm, you remind him that you need him to meet your needs.

Until you learn all about your husband's libido, including what makes it stronger and weaker, it would be best to assume he needs an orgasm at least once a day. Yes, that often. For some men, at some times, several times a day is what they need to be fully satisfied. Yes, that often. Although most men don't need orgasms that often most of the time.

> **Grandma Caroline:** *Having sex with your spouse frequently keeps them satisfied. Letting them go hungry for sex while away from home is like sending them to the grocery store when they're hungry for food... it makes them more susceptible to "impulse purchases." My husband wants to be faithful, and I want to make it*

*as easy as possible for him to do so, so I do my best to
keep his sex drive satisfied.*

Sometimes a woman's sex drive is stronger than a man's, but for
most couples it's the husband who wants and needs sex most
frequently. So, what can you do to satisfy your husband's sex
drive when you aren't in the mood? Grandma Synthia
recommends giving him a *quickie*, as described in the next
section.

Likewise, when you're on your period, your sex drive may
decline or temporarily stop, but his won't. So, you can deal with
it by laying on top of an adult disposable diaper to catch the
blood while in the missionary position, you can have sex in the
shower, or you can skip vaginal intercourse until your blood
flow slows down or stops. You have options, but you should not
make the decision without his consent. **It's very important
that you and your husband agree on how to keep both
your sex drives satisfied all the time.** If you hate the idea
of having intercourse while on your period, you may sometimes
need to put aside your concerns for your husband's sake or use
another alternative such as encouraging him to masturbate.

The same goes for when one of you is too ill to have sex. The
best solution may be to encourage your spouse to masturbate.
And that doesn't mean send them into the closet.... it can very
endearing for a man or woman to be laying next to their spouse
while they relieve themselves.

By using sex to the best of your ability, you can help your
husband stay faithful to you, and help him have a positive
attitude toward life that will help him be successful. So, do your
best to let your husband give you orgasms, and keep your
husband's sex drive fully satisfied.

Mastering the Quickie

A *quickie* is having sexual activity for the purpose of getting
either you or your husband to an orgasm as quickly as possible.

The Male Quickie

Men benefit from foreplay as much as women, but a quickie
won't allow time for more than a smidgen of that. If you want to
give your husband an orgasm as quickly as possible, get into his
pants and get your mouth on his penis. Alternate between
moving your head up and down to change the depth and then

swirling your tongue over the head of his penis. Nothing will give him an erection faster than that. If you're giving him a quickie because he's already got a hard-on, you can skip this.

As soon as he's hard, get him inside you and whoever's on top needs to get moving so that his erection is thrusting in and out of you. Most of the time, this will be your vagina, but it could be any alternative, such as anal or mammary (breast).

Now if you really want this to work, the best way is for you to put on a show. Basically, you have to fake a buildup to an orgasm of your own.

If he's healthy, that's all it takes, most of the time. If his penis becomes soft before he reaches an orgasm, quickly put it in your mouth until it gets hard again, and then resume intercourse and your show.

About Faking

Faking is bad, but fake-faking is good!

Faking is being deceptive. That's when you're faking and your spouse doesn't know you're faking. Because sooner or later, they're going to find out you've been faking and feel deceived. And they'll feel deceived because they *were* deceived, and the trust between you will have suffered, perhaps permanently. From then on, they may never be completely sure if you're faking or not, and that's a big turn-off.

In contrast, fake-faking is a game, a pretense, in which the spouse who's faking makes it obvious that they're faking. How do you make it obvious? The best way is to say so. "Honey, I'm going to pretend to be getting close to an orgasm while we have a quickie, to try to help you cum as quickly as you can." Anything to make it clear your pretending. You won't always need to make a statement, however. It won't be long, and you and your husband will develop an instinct for a set of unspoken clues you each give when one of you is "performing".

So, how should you perform? **Moan and move.**

Moan a lot, and build up your moaning as your husband builds toward a climax. If you use sexy talk, that should be part of your performance, starting light and becoming more and more explicit and emphatic.

Note that the closer a person gets to an orgasm, the less their higher brain functions work, so your husband may not easily be aware of talk when you're giving him directions. If you ask him to let you turn over, for instance, you may have to say it several times for it to sink in. Or you could just roll over, and let him adjust, which he may do subconsciously.

Maximizing your performance will require movement on your part. If you're on top or otherwise in control, you'll be doing most of the movement, but even if you're lying in a missionary position you need to move a little bit in order to enhance the pretense that you're building to an orgasm. Moan while you move to show that the movement is a sensual movement instead of an attempt to alleviate a discomfort (even if it is). Even very subtle movements can be all that's needed when accompanied by moaning. A small movement in your legs, your hips, or running your fingers over his skin or through his hair can have a powerful effect.

When you're pretending, don't build up too fast. If you sound like you're about to move the Earth the moment he penetrates you, it will be too inconsistent with reality to feed into his passion and you won't be able to notch it up. Try to time the increases in your performance to coincide with your husband's level of excitement.

Finally, when he reaches an orgasm, you can have a big impact on the quality of that orgasm by pretending to have an orgasm of your own at the same time.

Sometimes, even when you're husband thought you were pretending, your performance will be so good he may ask you if in fact you really had an orgasm that time. **Always be honest.** Unless you did, which is extremely unlikely when giving a quickie, tell him that you didn't actually have an orgasm, but that you very much enjoyed feeling him move inside you, feeling him ejaculate inside you, watching his face as he came, etc. If you really didn't enjoy anything that time, tell him that no, you really didn't feel all that great, but that he's made you feel so great in the past it's easy for you to replay those experiences for him.

If you're always honest, his only doubts will be wondering how he was so fortunate to get a wife as exceptional as you!

The Female Quickie

Most women don't want quickies as often as men do. In fact, they usually want a lot of buildup – with as much romance, ambiance, and tenderness as possible. But for many women, there are a few times when you're just plain aching for an orgasm and *want it now*.

For those times, you need to ask your husband for a quickie. Don't waste time and frustration waiting for him to figure it out. He won't. So tell him. As clearly as possible.

And until he becomes well practiced at what things help you get to an orgasm the quickest, you may have to tell him exactly what to do. If you don't know, the two of you have a lot of experimenting to do.

For most women, a successful quickie will require some variation of clitoral stimulation *for as long as it takes*. The vast majority of the time, that means his tongue on your clit, not his fingers. For some women, a steady stroking is best, and for others, a constantly increasing frequency is best (start slow, get faster and faster). And for many women, variety is necessary, using one technique one time, then another technique the next time.

Here are Grandma Synthia's recommendations for things to try:
- Husband lying on top of you with his crotch above or near your face while licking your clitoris, putting his torso over your breasts.
- Husband lying between your legs while licking your clitoris, reaching up to massage a breast.
- Husband lying between your legs while licking your clitoris and inserting one or more fingers into your vagina and/or anus.
- Husband lying between your legs while licking your clitoris and using toys in your vagina and/or anus.
- A hump-rub with you lying face up and your husband penetrating your vagina from a kneeling position while you massage your clitoris.

Note: When you're husband's licking you, he can't be talking at the same time. For a few women, hearing loving talk from their husband is necessary to achieve an orgasm, so for them, an option that keeps their husband's tongue free, such as the hump-rub, is very important.

Note: For your quickie, when in a "69" position, don't put your mouth on your husband's penis unless it increases *your* level of excitement. Your quickie is all about *your* orgasm.

Mild Warning: A female quickie often gets the husband so aroused that *he'll* need a quickie immediately after. Fortunately, that works out well for the many women who like the feel of penetration immediately after an orgasm, especially one that was induced by cunnilingus.

> ***Grandma Kelly:*** *All men like oral sex, I suspect, but most women* <u>need</u> *oral sex. I was a lesbian as a teenager and through most of my twenties, and I was physically intimate with many other women, and that almost always meant licking each other's clits as the primary activity. Most of us enjoyed other sexual activities, but would not have been able to reach an orgasm if not for direct massage of our clitorises, and nothing felt better than a talented tongue. On the rare occasions when men were discussed, it was usually to complain about early attempts to have heterosexual relationships, and how the men were universally selfish, incompetent, or both. We all assumed that it required a woman to really know how to satisfy a woman.*
>
> *After I became a Christian, I remained with the partner I had been with for over a year, but she began to despise my faith and eventually she left me. I was alone for a long time but still considered myself a lesbian Christian. Then one day I thought about that and wondered if I shouldn't be a Christian lesbian instead. That question led me into soul-searching and Bible study, and I finally concluded, very reluctantly, that I should never again practice homosexuality. That was depressing, because I thought it meant a life alone or a very sexually frustrating marriage.*
>
> *Well, I eventually fell in love with a wonderful man, and thought marriage to him would be worthwhile despite sexual frustration. But I was also afraid that I was being too optimistic due to "being in love". Nevertheless, when he proposed, I accepted, we set a date, and the date approached.*
>
> *A few weeks before the wedding, a meeting was arranged with one of my future Grandmothers-in-law.*
>
> *Wow, did she have a lot to teach me about sex! I was too stunned to remember much of it, but one thing*

stood out. Grandma said her husband performed cunnilingus as often as she wanted, <u>as long as she wanted</u>, usually without her asking, about every other day!

Shortly after that, my husband-to-be and I had some very frank pre-marriage discussions based on a guidebook, and one discussion covered our sexual expectations. I was quite astonished to hear the man who was going to share my bed talk about how he was looking forward to tasting me and learning how to satisfy me in every possible way.

I should have been happy, of course, but the truth is I doubted. It was too good to be true. I doubted right up until our wedding night when he put his head between my legs for the first time. I cried, and he stopped, worried about me. Once I convinced him I was crying because I was happy, he resumed... and gave me reason to cry all night.

I had known physical satisfaction many times, with many people, but I had never before known the joy I experienced that night. And yes, a man can satisfy a woman as well as another woman can, if he's as considerate and capable as my husband!

Deep-Throating

Men love fellatio, especially deep-throating, which is when you insert his penis into your mouth past the epiglottis and into your throat (if your husband's penis is long enough). This will put your lips all the way up to his abdomen and testicles, and should be done with the wife in control, because you may not be able to breathe this way. Deep-throating can have the advantage of not having any semen to clean up if your husband ejaculates in your mouth, and if you deep-throat him while he ejaculates, you won't taste the semen because it's past your taste buds.

Most women have to practice to overcome their gag reflex when deep-throating.[25] The gag reflex is an involuntary muscle contraction at the back of your throat to prevent swallowing. Many women never overcome it, and many aren't even aware that it's possible, but in fact, your mind suppresses (or doesn't invoke) the gag reflex every time you swallow food or drink.

---

[25] In one study, 37% of healthy people didn't have a gag reflex, (http://www.ncbi.nlm.nih.gov/pubmed/7861875), and another study shows that in people who have a gag reflex, the sensitivity of the reflex varies (http://www.pubmedcentral.nih.gov/articlerender.fcgi?artid=486467).

If you're one of the majority who do have a natural gag reflex, you can do 3 things to reduce or eliminate it:

- Short-Term Desensitization
- Long-Term Desensitization
- Oral Sex Lubricant

You can quickly suppress your gag reflex with sprays that numb the back of the throat, such as "Comfortably Numb Deep Throat Spray," available in multiple flavors.

You can develop long-term suppression of your gag reflex by brushing the back of your tongue with your toothbrush (which also improves your breath). Brush far enough back until it feels uncomfortable, and keep doing it for a few minutes. It may take days, but you should eventually be able to brush in that spot without any discomfort. When you can, move the brush a little further back, and repeat until you can go all the way back.

Most adults know about using a personal lubricant for vaginal or anal sex, but some lubricants (liquids and gels) are safe to swallow, and that means you can use them for oral sex. **Using an edible lubricant while deep-throating decreases the sensitivity of the gag reflex in many people.** If you want to try lubricants for oral sex, use water-based lubes that are edible, since you'll swallow some. They're available in many flavors, with some coming in sampler packs with a variety of flavors. Some are specifically marked as sugarless, in case you're sensitive to sugar (you shouldn't be swallowing enough for calories to be a problem). Make sure you do NOT use silicone-based or "stimulating" lubricants for oral sex. Some oil-based lubes are edible, but can be messier and harder to clean up.

Don't get discouraged if you fail the first few times you try to go from simple fellatio to deep-throating, or if you get your husband's penis all the way in and then panic. You may just need a lot more practice before you become comfortable with having his penis all the way in. When learning, use a kneeling position and use one or both hands to stroke any part of the shaft and head when it's not in your mouth. Alternate between attempts to take him all the way in with using your tongue to tickle the glans and frenulum, and lick up and down the entire shaft. Occasionally use one hand to fondle his testicles, perineum, anus, or P-spot while you keep your mouth busy at the same time.

If your husband is fortunate enough that you can learn to deep-throat him, expect a powerful reaction. **Men say deep-throating feels different from any other form of sex**, and they *love* it. And that's just from basic, get-it-all-the-way-in action. Once you're comfortable with that, there are a variety of ways you can enhance the effect and drive your man wild, such as in a 69 position. (If you fantasize about your husband being your love-slave, you may find that these techniques make your dream come true!) Try these techniques while his penis is fully inserted and your lips are against his abdomen and testicles:

- Humming: It's your own built-in deep-throat vibrator!
- Tonguing: Move your tongue forward and back, then side-to-side. You may not be able to move it a lot, but just a little will thrill him. Try to extend your tongue outside your mouth for an extra thrill for him.
- Head-Twisting: Tilt your head from side to side. Again, you won't be able to move your head a lot, but even a little will have a big impact.
- Swallowing: Make a "swallowing" action in the back of your throat. Swallowing is a muscular effort, and if you do this while his penis is back there, he'll love it.

Comfort Sex

If your spouse suffers an emotional upheaval, such as the death of a parent, or the loss of their job, sex can be an excellent emotional stabilizer. During such times try to give extra attention to their sex needs, which may include prolonged foreplay, a quickie, or anything in between.

Under such circumstances, you should expect that they may need an orgasm, but they may be poorly prepared to give one. However, the opposite may also be true: sometimes a person under great stress may derive more emotional fulfillment from giving an orgasm and have little desire to receive one.

Also, their sexual desires and needs may change from moment to moment, so you need to pay close attention to the subtle clues they give. It's also okay to simply ask them if they want sex, or how they want sex, but don't be surprised if they don't actually know what they want. They may say they don't want sex, but start kissing and a minute later be having intercourse with you.

Sensuality Improvement Guide

Sensuality in this book means how aware a person is of their sense of touch. That sense may be augmented by the other senses of sight, smell, taste, and hearing, but it primarily the sense of touch.

Everyone has a different level of strength in their sex drive, their libido, and it changes over time and with different circumstances. Likewise, while people are having sex, their level of sensuality may change, generally becoming more and more sensitive as a person builds toward an orgasm.

If you're happy with your level of sensuality but your spouse wants you to become more sensual, forget it. In that case, there's a problem with your spouse accepting you as you are, and not a problem with you. But sometimes a person isn't satisfied with their own sensuality and wants to improve it. The following suggestions are for those people:

- Focus on yourself alone. This is not the time to think about making your spouse feel good.
- Use only a sensual environment. Candlelight helps set the mood. Barking dogs don't.
- Decide on lotions and toys beforehand. This is not the time to be surprised.
- Have your spouse start touching you, or start touching yourself, or control your spouse's hands with your own.
- Begin touching in your least sensitive areas and as slowly as *you* want, more toward more sensitive areas. Touch *every* inch of your body.
- Use stroking touches, pressure touches, gentle squeezing, gentle sucking, and brushing fingers through hair.
- Increase touching as slowly as you want, but eventually your entire body should be touched.

> **Hot Sex Tip:** Want to have sex, but don't want to say so? Take your lover's hand and suck on one of their fingers while looking them in the eyes. If they have a pulse, they should get the message.

Pregnant Sex

Have all the sex you want while you're pregnant, in any position you want. **Sex will not hurt your baby, and you will not induce labor!** This is true even if you're carrying twins or triplets. (No one in Grandma's family has experience with more than triplets, but we suspect nothing's safe with four or more!)

Have all the orgasms you want, right up until your water breaks. **Having orgasms will not hurt your baby and will not induce labor!** In your last couple of months, you might pray for it to induce labor, but it won't.

Speaking of all-you-want, **your sex drive may change while you're pregnant** and your hormone levels fluctuate. When it goes up, no problem. Have fun! When they go down, though, remember you have a husband whose sexual needs will remain strong. Some men even find the pregnant female form so exotic that they're sexually stimulated more than usual.

Hopefully, your husband's heart is faithful to you, and will keep his body faithful no matter what, but you can **make it as easy as possible for him by getting him off as often as he needs it**.

Depending on what your favorite positions are, **you may have to experiment with new positions,** and you may have to get creative. Grandma strongly suspects Mr. & Mrs. Kama Sutra[26] discovered all those exotic positions while she was pregnant. When your belly gets big enough, the basic rule is for you to lie, sit, or recline in whatever position is most comfortable for you, and let your husband do whatever contortions it takes for him to find a way to penetrate you. For him to get his mouth on your clitoris, you'll need to cooperate a little more than that.

If you're ever having trouble having intercourse while pregnant because you can't find a comfortable position, or for any other reason, remember that **you and your husband have other options,** including fellatio, using your hands to get him off, or getting him started and encouraging him to get himself off beside you instead of inside you. We say it elsewhere in this book, but we'll repeat it here. The most emotionally intimate thing a man or woman can do with their spouse is masturbate in front of them.

---

[26] No, that's not anyone's real names.

Moving on, **there's one major advantage to sex while pregnant:** you don't need any birth control! Seriously, if condoms are your usual means of birth control, your husband won't have to use them while you're pregnant, and the increased sensuality he experiences may make him a lot more eager for sex than usual.

There's another advantage to sex while pregnant: your husband may usually expect your undivided attention while he's thrusting inside you, even if you're not aroused. When you're pregnant, though, he's likely to be far more accommodating of some little eccentricities like you watching television and eating ice cream while he bangs away. Grandma's leading theory for this is that the husband is so grateful to keep getting sex, that he'll put up with anything rather than encourage you to use the pregnancy as an excuse to opt-out of sex.

On a more serious note, **if you keep your husband's sex drive satisfied throughout your pregnancy,** it can increase his long-term appreciation of you *immeasurably*. For a man, it's one thing to have a devoted wife who loves him, but it's on another level entirely to have a devoted wife who loves him and works at keeping him sexually fulfilled, even when its most inconvenient and least desirable to her.

Nipple Conditioning

Okay, you're pregnant, and in a few months you're going to have a baby. That baby will probably want to eat. You've got two choices: baby formula or breast milk. Almost everyone agrees that breast milk is better for the baby. It's also natural and free. Natural, though, doesn't necessarily mean easy.

Some women have an easy time breastfeeding with no preparation. For others, it can be quite painful and frustrating trying to get used to it. Your breasts can hurt and your hungry baby may be getting little milk, neither of which is an ideal situation. That's why many mothers give up quickly.

Well, you have 9 months while you're pregnant to get your nipples ready, and you have a training partner: your husband! You need to toughen up your tits, and it's better to make them hurt now than wait until your baby is starving and you're tempted to quit nursing and switch to formula. On the brighter side, conditioning your nipples can be erotic and fun, at least part of the time.

How do you condition your nipples? Sucking and squeezing. A lot. Your husband can suck them, and you can both squeeze them and rub them between your index finger and thumb.

When you start, light sucking and sexy squeezing won't hurt, but as you get closer and closer to your due-date, you need to start sucking and squeezing *harder and harder*. Yes, hard enough to hurt. And you need to keep it up, even though it hurts. For awhile, it may seem like there's no end in sight to the pain and discomfort, but there is. **You can get to the point where your nipples can handle very hard sucking without pain.** And you can get to this level of conditioning *before* your baby's born.

There are two benefits to achieving this level of conditioning: you can nurse your baby successfully without pain, and... your nipples become a greater source of physical pleasure, before, during, and after sex! So, train hard, persevere, and reap the benefits for years to come!

Sex After Children

What changes are there in your sex life after you have your first child? You have less time for sex and you have less energy for sex.

What changes are there in your sex life after you have each additional child? You have much less time for sex and you have much less energy for sex.

There are some couples who decide not to have children because they don't want to decrease their sexual activities or because they don't want to lower their standard of living (children are expensive). Don't give these folks a hard time... the world is now filled with people, and we don't need every couple to procreate.

On the bright side, having children doesn't mean you stop having sex. You just have to adapt a little. Well, okay, you have to adapt a lot. Here are some recommendations for adapting your sex life when there are children in the house that are old enough that you want to hide your sexual activities...

Time: Sometimes your kids are all at school, but unfortunately, that's usually when we're at work. Mostly you'll need to have sex when the kids are asleep or all away from home for a little while at sleepovers at friends' houses, at a movie theater, etc.

Scheduling sex might not seem very adventurous or romantic, but don't dismiss the idea without trying it. It can work extremely well, as your anticipation builds toward the appointed date and time.

Energy: Parents often have less energy for sex, perhaps because they're a little older, or because they have so many more things to do. If you've had a busy day, try to relax a little while before bedtime if you want to have sex when you go to bed. Weekends are usually a lot better energy-wise, unless you fill up your schedule too heavily driving kids all over the place. Limiting how much you allow your children to convince you to do can mean more energy for sex later.

Sound: Sex can be noisy, so you'll have to learn how to lower the volume or wait until they're sound asleep. Until they hit their late teens, most kids do sleep soundly, even if they sometimes take awhile to get to sleep. You can move your headboard away from the wall a bit so it stops banging, you might get a new mattress or box springs that doesn't squeak so much, and you might want to restrain your moaning or use a gag. Seriously. Lots of folks don't realize just how loud they get when they have an orgasm. You might want to record yourself from outside your bedroom and play it back just to check.

Most likely, your kids will eventually hear you having sex. It's okay. They'll learn that sex really is normal when they realize that even their parents do it!

Away From Home: Sometimes when you can afford it, you can hire a baby-sitter for an evening to go out on a date. There's no reason that date can't include sex, either in the car, at a cheap motel, or once in awhile at a nice hotel. If you can't afford to hire a good baby-sitter, you might be able to trade baby-sitting services with another couple. Swapping with other couples is also a good way to have overnight baby-sitters. Your friends can baby-sit your kids at their house and you can have sex at home, or they can stay at your house and you can have sex in a motel or hotel. And for the outdoorsy folks, a double sleeping bag and camping tent might do just fine.

Hiding Books and Toys: A book on the Kama Sutra may not be something you want your 9-year-old to stumble across. Likewise if you have specialized sex toys like a vibrating cock ring or a strap-on anal dildo. The best thing to keep them from prying eyes is to get a small lock box and keep it locked. Sooner or later, your kids are likely to find the box and if they weren't intentionally snooping, they may ask what's in it or why it's locked. Until they're old enough to understand, just tell them it's some personal things just for Mommy and Daddy.

Sex Education: Children grow up. And there are a lot of twisted people who would harm your children sexually as well as in other ways. So you protect them as well as you can. Eventually, they begin to become more and more independent of your protections. And they might fall in love with a person who tries to pressure them into sex. That person may not know that they already have the HIV virus, or any of many other sexual diseases, or they may be so twisted that they don't care. What is true love to your child may be an insignificant fling to the person they've set their heart on.

You can't protect your children from everything all the time. But if you want to do your best against the most likely dangers they'll face in life, you need to educate them the entire time they're growing up. Teach them about both sex & morality, at whatever level is appropriate for their ages. And when your children are ready to get married, we hope you consider giving them a copy of this book to help prepare them for marriage.

Senior Sex

Being old doesn't mean malfunctioning, and that's not what Senior Sex is about. *For sex despite disabilities and other problems, see the Alternative Sex and Problems Affecting Sex sections that follow.*

If you have sex less frequently as you get older, as most people do, that doesn't mean that it becomes less fulfilling. On the contrary, **after decades of building trust and exploring each other's needs and abilities, sex can be even more fulfilling**. Some adaptation may be necessary, such as using more lubricant after a woman goes through menopause.

Sex problems may not be an inevitable part of the aging process, but may result from specific emotional or physical health problems, or from relationship problems. In one large study of 57-to-85 year old men and women, about half reported at least one problem interfered with their sex lives in the past 12 months. The good news is that about half had no problems!

The overall results indicate that senior women are more likely than senior men to have problems due to current or previous urinary tract problems or due to current or previous sexually transmitted diseases (STD). A previous STD increases the chance that a senior woman will have pain during intercourse by about 400%, and increases the chance of lubrication problems by about 300%. If this ever applies to you, just use plenty of lubricant!

The most common physical problem for senior men is erectile dysfunction (ED), which makes it difficult or impossible to achieve or maintain an erection. Medication or surgery can often help with ED. A previous STD increases the chance of not sensing any pleasure from sex by about 500%.

For both men and women, the most common mental problem, by far, is performance anxiety. Men who were married or widowed were half as likely as their divorced or separated counterparts to suffer from performance anxiety.

In other studies, and in many anecdotal stories from within Grandma's family, many medications can cause temporary sexual problems.

There are also many medications and medical procedures that can help seniors compensate for sexual problems, and these should be investigated by consulting a physician.

Alternative Sex

Most of the time a husband and wife don't want to have sex. Okay, don't. Many times a husband and wife will both want to have sex. So do it. And often, only one member of a couple will be in the mood, so either they have to wait to satisfy their sex drive, or masturbate, or their spouse has to cooperate even though they aren't interested for their own sake.

But then there are times when a husband or wife wants to have sex, but can't due to physical or emotional limitations. There can also be times when your sex drive is telling you to have sex, but you'd really rather that your sex drive just shut up and leave you alone. For these kinds of conditions, Grandma offers some advice on having ¾ sex, tenderness sex, and sex hibernation...

¾ Sex

How do you "have sex" with someone who is not physically capable? Someone who is missing sex organs, is immobile while recovering from serious injury or illness, is hypersensitive to touch, etc.?

Couples can be very creative when necessary, and if one spouse can't move very well, there are often ways to get both husband and wife to orgasm with only one person doing all the work. That's great, but that's not ¾ sex. Grandma considers "whole" sex as both husband and wife having an orgasm. By this measure, if one spouse doesn't want to have sex and the other masturbates without assistance, that's ½ sex. Often ½ sex is satisfactory to both spouses, but when both are up to it, whole sex is nicer, we think.

If one spouse helps the other reach an orgasm without reaching one of their own, that spouse has participated in sex without having an orgasm, and we describe the actions of that spouse alone as ¼ sex. Looking at the sexual episode for both husband and wife, one has an orgasm (½ sex) and the other contributes to that orgasm but doesn't have an orgasm of their own (¼ sex), so ½ sex plus ¼ sex = ¾ sex!

Any couple can have ¾ sex anytime they wish, but when a spouse is physically incapable of having an orgasm, ¾ sex may be the best they can achieve.

Selfish people may not derive any pleasure from helping a spouse achieve an orgasm if they feel no sexual pleasure themselves, but we hope that's extremely rare. Marriage is all about loving each other and caring about the other's needs, not about having a permanent partner to trade orgasms. Grandma has several stories from within our family about relationships limited to ¾ sex where both husband and wife reports high levels of sexual satisfaction and overall marital happiness.

Here's a powerful story compiled from several of Grandma Victoria's daughters and granddaughters:

> **Grandma Victoria:** *I was born in 1907 and married "Victor" in 1930. We were farmers, and didn't use*

contraception because it was normal for farming families to want as many kids as they could have. Life was hard sometimes, but we were blessed with 7 children, 6 of whom lived to become adults. Farm life kept us pretty tired most of the time, but we still managed to enjoy sex, and Vic got pretty good at giving me orgasms on Saturday nights.

At the time the United States became involved in World War II in 1942, our family farm wasn't prospering, and Victor decided to join the military. He might have been able to get an exemption from the draft due to being a farmer, but he felt it wasn't fair since our farm was producing so little, and besides that, he also expected Army pay to be dependable. Vic had most of his pay sent home, and he ended up fighting in France. During one skirmish, he was severely wounded by a grenade and by several bullets. If there had been many casualties at the time, he probably wouldn't have survived, but several doctors were able to give him a lot of attention, and eventually they were able to send him home. He was alive, but he had no legs, no penis, no testicles, and little use of his arms, which were in almost constant pain.

We were thrilled to have him home alive, despite his disabilities, and the kids and I all took pride in waiting on our beloved war hero hand-and-foot, and pushing his wheelchair. Victor, though, had a lot of trouble trying to adjust.

He was tormented by the death of one of our children while he was away, thinking that those fateful events wouldn't have happened if he hadn't enlisted. He was also besieged with terrible nightmares about the war almost every night. And if that wasn't enough, he was now in a situation in which everyone was helping him and he wasn't able to help anyone else.

One night, in tears, Victor told me he wanted to die, that he just couldn't endure the suffering any longer. That broke my heart, and I begged him not to do anything rash, and I began praying more earnestly that I ever had before.

Since Victor had first come home, I knew that sex wasn't possible, as I was the one who emptied his bowel and bladder bags and bathed him in bed or in his chair. I had gotten used to not having sex while he was still overseas, and not having sex after he came home hadn't bothered me at all. But we hadn't talked about it, either.

GREAT SEX

On another night when Victor was despondent, he talked and talked, including lamenting all the things he missed. One of the things he said he missed the most was giving me kicks (what he called my orgasms because of the way my legs always shook). I noticed he didn't say he missed having orgasms himself, just that he very much missed giving me orgasms. After awhile, I asked if he'd like to try. He just cried and nodded.

I wasn't sure what we could do, and was afraid that a disappointment would be devastating to him, but I got out of bed to wash up at the basin while I thought up ideas. And the first idea I had was to stop. I lit the lamps (we still didn't have electric lights) and put Vic's glasses on him, and moved the basin stand close to the bed as I had done many times to bathe him. This time, though, I slowly undressed in front of my beloved, and I think it would be fair to say he stared in awe. Normally, I wouldn't bathe completely naked, I'd just bathe one exposed part at a time. This time, though, I stood with nothing on as I slowly and tenderly washed my body for my lover. Vic was gasping and moaning encouragement and thanks.

When I had finished bathing, I left one lamp lit, put Vic's glasses away, and pulled him lower in the bed. I crawled onto him, until my nub was right over his mouth.

It wasn't a position we had ever used before, but when his familiar tongue touched me again, I couldn't last a minute. I had the best orgasm of my life.

It was actually funny, because I lost control of myself, but I knew I was on top of his face and was afraid of smothering him, so I struggled to roll off as quickly as I possibly could. When I did, I rolled right off onto the floor! And I was still too overcome to be able to move much or even talk, so Vic started to panic that something was horribly wrong with me and started to yell for help while I was stark naked on the floor!! Fortunately, I recovered enough before help arrived to keep them from bursting into the room. We were able to get everyone to go back to bed without answering any questions, but the next day, answers were demanded. Vic and I told the tale (without all the details), and everyone howled with laughter.

Also the next day, the change in Victor was dramatic. He sounded better, he looked better, he looked stronger, he looked healthier, his constant pain seemed to bother him a lot less, and he was able to push his wheelchair a lot more by himself. He was happy.

And for the first time since he had been home, he was optimistic about life.

From then on until he passed away, every Saturday night I mounted my loving husband, and he licked me into a state of bliss. Even after diabetic retinopathy took his eyesight, Victor still took great pleasure in giving me more pleasure than one woman could ever deserve.

Whenever Grandma Victoria would tell her tale to a granddaughter, even when she was old and frail, she would get a big smile on her face, and say how she could still remember that one orgasm as if it were yesterday.

And that was the gift of a man who was unable to have an orgasm of his own.

Tenderness Sex

How do you have sex with someone who is very delicate emotionally? Very tenderly.

People can suffer from any of a huge variety of problems that include emotional struggles, such as anxiety, bipolar disorder, schizophrenia, substance abuse, etc. Often these folk are able to have normal sex, and it can sometimes boost their mental state just like it might boost anyone else's.

However, there may be times when an emotionally disturbed spouse's sex drive may be demanding sexual activity but their mental condition just isn't up to the job. For those times, the best solution might not be to avoid sex altogether, but to try very low-grade sex, or what Grandma calls *tenderness-sex*.

You might think of tenderness-sex as extended foreplay, without escalating to intercourse. It can be in bed or anywhere, with or without clothes, and involves lots of kissing, caressing, and intimate touching. The goal is not orgasm, the goal is spending time together being intimate.

You might also think of tenderness-sex as a level below tantric sex. In tantric sex (not associated with Tantric Buddhism), intercourse and related activities are maintained as long as possible, while orgasms are avoided or postponed as long as possible in order to maximize the enjoyment of the pre-orgasmic plateau phase. In tenderness-sex, intercourse may not be included, but even if it is, physical pleasure is not the goal, emotional caring is the goal.

Important: If a doctor recommends a behavior-reward treatment for behavioral modification therapy, use something other than sex, such as a special meal, or a special trip to a favorite place. **Always give sex to your spouse freely and unconditionally, never as a reward.**

Sex Hibernation

What do you do with your sex drive if you end up alone? Sex drives don't turn off when your spouse dies or divorces you. What do you do with that annoying hunger?

You have several choices, but only two of them are good ones: Masturbate or Hibernate. This book has a whole chapter on masturbation, so we won't rehash that here. This is where we'll tell you how you can try to make your sex drive become dormant.

Notice we said *try*. This is much easier said than done. Often it's easier for women to put their sex drives into hibernation than it is for men. And it's often easier for older folks than younger folks. Are you seeing a pattern? **How easy it is to get your libido to hibernate depends on how strong your libido is.** And if a libido is very strong, it can be extremely difficult to switch it off. On the other hand, if your libido is very weak, you may not need to do anything... if you never want sex – your sex drive is already dormant.

Okay, you have a strong sex drive, you've been widowed or divorced, and you don't want to masturbate, you just want to forget about sex. You've got to take this very seriously if you want to have a real chance of success. Here are Grandma Synthia's suggestions:

Stay *very* busy. Very, very busy.

Avoid sexual thoughts. When you catch yourself heading in that direction, or find yourself well down that road, stop and find something else to focus on. Ladies, this means no romance.

Including no romantic thoughts, because romantic thoughts easily lead to sexual thoughts.

Sanitize the house. Get rid of all sex toys and sex books in the house. Get rid of all porn, including novels with even slightly racy scenes. Don't buy or borrow any books that have any possibility of having romantic or sexual scenes. We hate this next advice, but we have to include it because it really is important: Don't watch television. At all. These days, even the "news" often has sexual titillation.

Exercise. If you can make regular exercise a habit, it can help you become physically fatigued so that you get to sleep easier.

Never let your guard down. If you succeed, you may have worked very hard for it. If you don't want to inadvertently lose what you've gained, then you must work to keep it. Staying dormant requires constant vigilance.

Here's the worst news: If you start having success at avoiding sexual thoughts, it gets harder. Let's say an *icon* is a symbol that has specific ideas associated with it. The further you distance yourself from blatantly sexual icons, the more tempting moderately sexual icons become. And the further you get from moderate sexual icons, the more tempting innocent, non-sexual icons become.

Men who stop masturbating for days or weeks are very likely to start experiencing occasional wet dreams, which involve very erotic dreams that lead to a real-world ejaculation. The ejaculation usually causes the man to wake up, interrupting the dream, but bringing them to wakefulness with snippets of memory of the erotic dream. This can feel like a complete failure, and it can be tempting to give up and resume regular masturbation. If, however, you just chalk it up to your body making adjustments to a new sex-free conscious life, then it may become less of a problem as time goes by.

What if you succeed and decide you want to wake up your sex drive? If you fall in love and want to get married again, that's great. Get married and kick your sex drive into high gear! If you don't have any physical problems, turning your libido back on should be easy and natural. In fact, it will almost certainly happen without thinking about it at all, as soon as you let romance fill your heart again.

Problems Affecting Sex

Abuse: No form of abuse will exist in a healthy relationship, and no form of abuse should be tolerated in a relationship. Sexual or other physical abuse, and verbal or other mental/emotional are huge danger signs. If you abuse your spouse, leave them and get professional help, and do not ask to return until your abuse is completely under control. If you spouse is abusive to you, leave them immediately and take your children. If the danger is severe and immediate, go directly to the police and ask for help in getting into a safe house. Otherwise seek the support of family, friends, or your Church or other religious organization. Do not wait until the abuse becomes a fatal tragedy.

Anger: An inability or unwillingness to control anger will certainly not get a person's spouse in the mood to have sex. If you have this problem, see a physician, psychologist, anger-management counselor, or all of them.

Anxiety: Worrying about your ability to satisfy your spouse is a big issue for some people. The most important approach to dealing with this is communication. That's right, talk. Open and honest talking and listening by both spouses. Even if you think the primary problem is physical, with good communication, you may learn that it's not as big a deal as you thought. For example, if the husband can't get an erection, he may worry mightily that his wife will feel deprived, but once they talk it out, he may learn that she's not bothered by that at all as long as his tongue still works. Maybe you're scared your husband will think you look hideous if you have a breast removed, but if you talk about your fears, you may learn that he only cares about your health and that it's your smile that turns him on. For most physical and mental issues, there are solutions or workarounds, but they may not overcome anxiety by themselves if you don't talk it over.

Erectile Dysfunction (ED): ED may be caused by anxiety, disease, or by medications. It may also be relieved by medications, but the relieving medications may cause other side effects. If the problem is that he doesn't stay hard long enough, sometimes switching back and forth between fellatio and intercourse can keep him going. There are also penile implants that can solve some ED problems.

Diminished Sex Drive (Libido): If you think your libido is too low, it is. If you think your spouse's libido is too low but they're content with it, it's you have a problem with expectation, not your spouse having a libido problem. If you have a problem, there are ways to try to boost a sex drive that don't involve a prescription medication: aerobic exercise, relaxation techniques, using more variety in your sex practices, dietary/herbal supplements (e.g. choline, vitamin B5, or ginkgo biloba), or the use of arousing scents, such as musk. If none of these work, testosterone patches *may* increase the sex drive in men or women, but side effects are still being studied for therapeutic use.

Inability to Reach Orgasm: This may be physical or psychological, and you should seek professional help. First, though, check your current medications and see if this is a known side-effect. If so, you might ask your doctor to try replacing that medication with a different one.

Lack of Pleasure From Sex: This may be physical or psychological, and you should seek professional help. Like the above problem, first check your current medications for known side-effects.

Pain During Intercourse: This may be physical or psychological, and you should seek professional help. Like the above problem, first check your current medications for known side-effects.

Reaching Orgasm Too Quickly: (last time...) This may be physical or psychological, and you should seek professional help. Like the above problem, first check your current medications for known side-effects.

Vaginal Dryness: Generous use of personal lubricant will overcome most dryness issues, and the stimulating or flavored kinds can even enhance some activities. If they don't work, see a physician or psychologist.

Hidden Treasure:

You can trim your pubic hair with scissors while sitting on a toilet and the hair falls right in. This can make it much easier for your spouse to get their tongue where you like it, without making their tongue have to plow through a forest, and without the itchy side-effects of shaving. However, it usually doesn't itch to shave just a tiny patch, and you can use that to create a little design that only you and your lover know about.

WILD SEX

Remember the goals of this book? To help you enjoy sex and keep your husband satisfied. The chapter on Great Sex may be all you and your husband need, but as you get older, you may find that it becomes a little more difficult to move from the plateau stage to an orgasm. Some simple variety can spice things up a lot, and help you push your spouse over the edge of that plateau! The purpose of this chapter is to help stir your imagination and consider some options to fire-up your husband and yourself.

To be clear, some couples are happily married their entire adult lives and never practice any of the activities we think of as being on the wilder side of sexual play, and that's fine! If, however, you find it more difficult to get to an orgasm, or notice that it's more difficult for your husband, you might want to least try these additional ideas at least once, or once in a while.

How do we define wild? (Besides writing an explicit sex advice book?) As anything that would surprise basic-sex-only people if they knew you behaved that way. If you're married, everyone assumes you have sex, and if you have children, they know you have sex. Most people, though, will assume you have *basic* sex. But if you were to play a game of truth or dare at a baby shower and you were to confess to the other women that you have a French maid's outfit for sex fantasies with your husband, would they be at least mildly surprised? That's what we have in mind with these topics:

- Cheating With Your Husband
- Costumes
- The Appeal Of Heels
- Edgy Locations
- Sex Talk
- Grandma's Ooo-aah Club
- Sex Tech
- Advanced Sex Fantasy

Cheating <u>With</u> Your Husband

After awhile, the initial rush of falling in love, planning a wedding, getting married, having a honeymoon and getting adjusted to married life begins to melt into something of a routine. Many couples, if not most, are fine with that for their entire lives, but sometimes some people get bored and long again for the excitement of falling in love. Grandma Synthia suspects that's the primary reason some people have adulterous affairs.

Well, Grandma has a solution to regain some of those feelings without betraying your spouse. Go ahead and have an affair... with your husband!

Plan to meet at a restaurant, bar, or store you've never been to before and just happen to meet your husband, pretending you've never met each other before. Tease and flirt with each other. Then confide that you're bored with your spouse, and open to finding someone who might get your motor running again. Then... decide not to do anything about it and start to leave. But... turn at the last moment for a quick kiss that lasts a little too long, then rush away. Think about the encounter a day or two. Then go back to the same place hoping to see the other person again. And you do! And it turns out he only came hoping to find you. You look deeply into each other's eyes, and one of you points out that there's a hotel nearby...

Get the idea? You can use any of a million variations on this theme to stir your pot! And don't forget the little gifts that lovers give each other. Just make sure you keep them a secret from your husband. Wait, is that the real husband who's pretending he's not, or the pretend husband who's pretending he is, or...

Costumes

Costumes are *not* necessary in order to pretend, but they can enhance our ability to imagine and add a little fun. You can purchase or make elaborate costumes, but **just a simple token can do a lot to help set the mood**, and tokens are easier to hide from your kids. If you have a full suit of armor in your closet, your kids will definitely find that, but if you have a walking stick to use as a knight's sword, that's easier to explain.

Here are some of our favorite tokens and costumes:
- Grandma Anne likes her husband to wear a **tool belt** and nothing else. At other times, she'll wear it.
- Grandma Brenda uses an **apron** to turn herself into a maid.
- Grandma Caroline uses a TV **remote control** to control her husband's sexual activity.
- Grandma Elizabeth uses a **book** to turn into a magician casting sex spells on her hubby.
- Grandma Heather and her husband use plain **masks** to pretend they're having sex with strangers.
- Grandma Jennifer or her husband don a **bathroom towel** as a cape to become a superhero whose special power is giving orgasms.
- Grandma Kelly uses **exercise equipment** to become a (very) personal trainer.
- Grandma Lilly uses a **burqa** to become a Woman of Mystery.
- Grandma Rachael couldn't narrow it down to just one favorite. Some of her current favorites are a **tail** (attached to a little belt, and not wearing anything else, turns her into many kinds of animals), a **feather** in her hair (turns her into an Indian princess), **wigs**, a set of **strap-on wings** (explained to their children as a sentimental leftover from a costume in a high-school play, which it was), **toy handcuffs** (kept in a lock box with her sex toys), and a **dog collar** for her husband (also kept in lock box, and used with their dog's leash).
- Grandma Yvette uses a **miniskirt** to become a *full-service* waitress.

The Appeal of Heels

High heeled shoes are sexy. Most men think so and many if not most women think so. Pornographic videos frequently have women in heels, and often *only* in heels.

Why are heels sexy? There's no precise answer to that question, but here are some possibilities:
- It's mildly exotic. That is, it's not an everyday thing for most women.
- It's a subtle sexual signal. The signal could be from how it realigns a woman's hips, and/or from how it raises a

woman's crotch to be closer to the same height as a man's crotch, when standing.

- It's become a traditional symbol. It's sexy because everyone thinks it's sexy.

Grandma recommends that you avoid walking in high heels because infrequent walking in heels makes it dangerous as far as twisting an ankle, and too much of it will change your skeletal alignment. There are women who walk in heels most of the time, however, and prefer it, so if you fall into that camp, more power to you.

Even if you never *walk* in heels, you can still *wear* heels – in the bedroom. You can wear them only in bed... seriously. Get a cheap, pretty pair and try it and see if it turns your man on. Or, you can wear them while standing at the foot of the bed and leaning over it. Doing so will raise your vagina a few inches and change its angle, and depending on your respective heights, it can make a big difference in your husband's ability to penetrate you from behind, and can change the sensation for both of you.

Edgy Locations

Public and semi-private locations for sex can increase excitement while having sex, due to the novelty or the idea that you could be seen. Note that it doesn't mean being in a place where it's actually possible to be seen, although that would probably be exciting, but just the idea of it can be stimulating.

For example, if you're camping outdoors in a tent, no one can see you. With your eyes closed, however, you can easily hear the sounds of nature and imagine that there's no tent at all. If you're in a busy campground and other campers are still talking around the fire, that can make it seem like a public place.

If fact, you can have sex in many places outdoors even without a tent if the area is either dark, dense, or secluded enough.

Another place some couples find edgy is in a car. If you're parked in an isolated place, no one will be able to see you. If the windows are fogged up, no one will see regardless of where you park. (But remember to lock all the doors!) You can even have sex in the car while its parked in your garage and pretend it's in a public place, such as outside the grocery store.

You might also try having sex in front of a hotel window with the curtains open and the lights off, as long as there's no public balcony right outside that window. If you're in a sea-side hotel room and can open a window and turn off the air conditioning, you can have sex in bed while listening to the surf and pretending you're out on the beach.

Sex Talk

Grandma has three categories for sexy talk: romantic, explicit, and naughty.

Romantic talk is terms of endearment, such as "I love you", and "you're so beautiful", and they help initiate arousal or increase excitement.

Explicit talk uses precise terms to help give directions to your spouse, such as "take my clothes off", or "please lick my clit."

Naughty talk uses "bad" words and phrases to help initiate arousal or increase excitement, such as "eat me", or "hump me."

Grandma's not going to explain romantic talk in this book, because most readers will understand that without help. Some readers may need a little help in order to use explicit talk, so we'll present an Explicit Language Acclimation Guide next. Most readers will have doubts about using naughty language, so we'll discuss that, and then end this section with a couple of Naughty Language Acclimation Guides for those who want to try it but need help.

Explicit Language Acclimation Guide

The reason for this acclimation guide is to help those who need to use words and phrases they're initially too embarrassed to use. And it's important to use them to communicate clearly.

Please don't think that your spouse should know what you're thinking. God didn't give many people the ability to read minds. He did give most of us the ability to talk. Using it well may require you to use some or all of our Explicit Vocabulary at one time or another.

One of the most important things you can say is "that feels good". That's not too hard, right? Obviously it helps your spouse learn how make you feel good. But equally important, it tells your spouse that they have succeeded in a critical sexual ability, enhancing their own sexual self-esteem. However, while "that feels good" can be powerful, but it can be unclear when several things are going on at once. If you say, "that feels good", you may get a response of, "*what* feels good"? **It's important for both you and your spouse to be able to say exactly what you like, and what you don't like.**

To do so, follow these acclimation steps with the Explicit Vocabulary in order to become comfortable enough with it to use it when the time is right. You may be able to skip some steps, but if you really have difficulty saying these words out loud to your spouse, you may need to follow all these steps.

Repeat each step once a day until you become comfortable with that step.

1. Read the entire list to yourself.
2. When you're alone where no one can hear you, read the list out loud.
3. When you have some time alone in the bathroom and no one will be able to hear you, look at a word or phrase in the list, then look in the bathroom mirror as you say the word out loud. (It's okay if you blush or giggle!) Go through the whole list.
4. Repeat the list using trying different tones of voice (e.g. sultry, anxious, whisper, urgently).
5. When your spouse has also completed step 4, wait until you're together in bed and *without looking at each other*, take turns reading the list out loud.
6. When you're together in bed and *looking at each other*, take turns reading the list out loud in a plain voice.
7. When you're together in bed and *looking at each other*, take turns reading the list out loud in different tones of voice.
8. When you're together in the bedroom, take turns reading the list out loud, and each time you read a noun word or phrase, touch that part of your or your spouse's anatomy, and each time you read a verb or verb phrase, perform that action.
9. Make up some words or phrases of your own, such as "stuff my basket" as a euphemism for "come inside me", and jot them down here.
10. Repeat these steps using the Acclimation Phrases.

Explicit Vocabulary[27]

A-Spot	Anus
Arousal/aroused	Breast
Climax	Clit/clitoris
Condom	Cunnilingus
Ejaculate	Fellatio
Fingering	Foreplay
French Kiss	G-Spot
Head (*of penis*)	Intercourse
Lick	Lips (mouth)
Lips (vaginal)	Masturbation
Nipple	Orgasm
P-Spot	Penis
Perineum	Quickie
Scrotum	Semen
Shaft	Suck
Testicles	U-Spot
Vagina	

Acclimation Phrases[28]

Take my clothes off.
Take your clothes off.
Let me take your clothes off.
Touch my [*insert a noun*].
Kiss my [*insert a noun*].
Suck my [*insert a noun*].
I want your tongue on my [*insert a noun*].
Put your mouth on my [*insert a noun*].
I want your mouth on my [*insert a noun*].
I need your mouth on me.
Caress my breasts.

Suck my nipples.	That feels good.
That feels very good.	I want you to...
Spread your legs for me.	Spread your lips for me.
I need to come inside you.	I want to cum inside you.
Come inside me.	Fill me.
I need you inside me.	Penetrate me.
Let's mix some wine.	Water my garden.
A little more gently.	A little harder.
Go easier.	Do it harder.
Slow down.	Go faster.
Stop.	Don't stop.

---

[27] See the Glossary or the chapter on Basic Sex for definitions.
[28] Feel free to add "please" and other terms to these phrases.

Naughty Language

If you don't want to use any of these words, ever, that's okay. You can rip these pages out if you wish. But even if you have no intention of using such language any time soon, you might want to hang on to this in case you someday decide to try to use a naughty or semi-naughty word or phrase to surprise your spouse and a little spice to your routine.

One word can have different meanings, which may depend on the circumstances of its use. Some words that are wrong to use in one context may be acceptable in a different setting, or in a different manner, or at a different time.

Context Matters

If you're reluctant to use "dirty" talk in the bedroom when you first get married, that's fine! The kind of sexy talk you develop together with your husband should only be with your husband. If you both get used to it, it can be very arousing for your husband to hear you say "hump me", but you definitely shouldn't be saying that when anyone else is around.

Angry/Derogatory Usage vs. Sexy Usage

Some words that are wrong to use in one manner may be okay when used with a different intent. For example, the word "fuck" is still extremely offensive if shouted in anger as "fuck you!" But if you're honest, you'll have to admit the phrase has an entirely different meaning if uttered seductively by a wife to her husband as, "I'm going to fuck you until you can't stand up!"

The Rehabilitation Of Bad Words

In addition to different settings and different manner, time can also be a factor. Many "bad" words go through a progression from being considered very offensive to being considered completely inoffensive.

For example, in the 1970's "sucks" was only used as an exclamation as part of a phrase such as "he/she sucks dicks" or "sucks cocks", which was considered about as vile as anything that could be said. Then it morphed to being used as just "that sucks", but was still closely associated with the previous phrases and still considered extremely offensive. Over the intervening years, the association dimmed and has been almost lost, and even if it hadn't become disassociated, fellatio is no longer a disreputable topic. Today, "that sucks" is often used innocently as a euphemism for "that's too bad".

Another example is the word "fuck", which has been slang for sexual intercourse for hundreds of years. While it has been considered crude for most of that time, it has more recently lost some of its weight as an offensive word, perhaps due to its pervasive use in many R rated movies for its shock effect. Eventually such a shock value fades and the term may become much more common and less offensive.

The word "fuck", in particular, has the advantage of being a single syllable, which may be a reason why "fuck me" might be preferred over "please have sexual intercourse with me". People often prefer shorter words, especially in the heat of passion. However, the word "fuck" also has the disadvantage of being considered extremely bad for a very long time, and it's still too offensive for many Christians to bring themselves to utter, and most don't like to read it, either.

We Grandmas debated whether or not to include it, and weren't happy either way. Most of us *really* don't like it, but more than one of us most emphatically does like to use it in the bedroom. Eventually we decided to include it for 3 reasons: it has unmatched erotic power; younger people (our main intended audience is two generations younger than us) in general are not as bothered by it as we are; and because we originally set out to be as inclusive as possible of all sexual topics. We realize that some people may hate this book because it has this word in it, but we're guessing they're likely to hate it for many other reasons as well, so excluding one word wouldn't really help.

Naughty Language Acclimation

For most Christians and many others, getting comfortable using naughty words will be far more difficult than getting use to explicit words, even if it's only used with your spouse in a loving manner. That's okay. **You don't have to use any naughty words, ever,** so it certainly won't matter if it takes you a long time to become able to use some. Or, **you might like hearing your spouse use them** even if you don't want to say them.

If you decide you want to practice some of these words, but find others too offensive, that's fine! You can use a pencil and line through those if you want to.

Although getting use to naughty words can feel very awkward at first, you can get used to them if you persist past the awkward stage. That's what our acclimation guides are for.

And, of course, you can choose just to use one word. In fact, that's the basis of our first naughty language acclimation guide...

Slow-Start Naughty Language Guide

1. Pick a relatively mild word from the naughty vocabulary, such as "rack", which is slang for a woman's breasts.
2. When you're alone, practice using the word in sentences you could use with your spouse. The wife could plan to pose in her bra and say, "How do you like my rack?", or the husband could plan to caress his wife's breasts through her blouse while whispering, "You have a gorgeous rack." Repeat this step until you're comfortable with this word in private.
3. When you're alone with your spouse, use one of the sentences you practiced with your new naughty word. It's okay to be embarrassed at first, even extremely embarrassed. Just whisper it. Repeat this step until you're comfortable with this word in front of your spouse.
4. Start this list over with a new word. Over time, decide if you want to choose slightly more daring words.

Rapid-Start Naughty Lang. Guide

1. Read the entire list to yourself.
2. When you're alone where no one can hear you, read the list out loud.
3. When you have some time alone in the bathroom and no one will be able to hear you, look at a word or phrase in the list, then look in the bathroom mirror as you say the word out loud. It's okay if you blush or whisper, but go through the whole list.
4. Repeat the list using trying different tones of voice (e.g. sultry, anxious, whisper, urgently).
5. When your spouse has also completed step 4, wait until you're together in bed and *without looking at each other*, take turns reading the list out loud in a plain voice.
6. Still without looking at each other, take turns reading the list out loud in different tones of voice.
7. When you're together in bed and *looking at each other*, take turns reading the list out loud.

8. When you're together in the bedroom, take turns reading the list out loud, and each time you read a noun word or phrase, touch that part of your or your spouse's anatomy, and each time you read a verb or verb phrase, perform that action.
9. Repeat this list with the naughty phrases.

Naughty Vocabulary[29]

Ass	Balls
Bang	Beaver
Blow job	Boner
Bonk	Boobs
Bush	Cameltoe
Cherry	Cock
Cream	Cum
Cunt	Deep throat
Dick	Dong
Drill	Eating pussy
Fuck/Fucking	Get laid
Going down	Hard-on
Hooters	Horny
Hump / Humping	Jack-off
Jism	Jizz
Jugs	Knockers
Licking out	Melons
Muff	Nail
Nuts	Rack
Rocks	Tits
Titties	Plug
Pound / Pounding	Prick
Pussy	Screw / Screwing
Shag	Spooge
Spreading	Spunk
Strip	Suck / Sucking
Sucking off	Tail
Tent pole	Tits/Titties
Tit job	Tongue-fuck
Tool	

Phrases for Either Spouse to Say

I'm getting a little horny.
I'm getting really horny.
My socks are getting wet.
Fuck my ear with your tongue.

[29] See the Glossary for definitions.

Strip for me.	Strip.
Eat me.	Suck me.
Hump me.	Screw me.
Hump me.	Shag me.
Go down on me.	Lick me.
I want you to fuck me.	I want to fuck you.

Please fuck me *now*.
I'm going to fuck you until you can't stand up.
I'm going to ride you hard and put you up wet.
Suck my [*insert noun or noun phrase*]
Touch my [*insert noun or noun phrase*]
Stroke my [*insert noun or noun phrase*]

Phrases for a Husband to Say

Do you like my cock?
Do you want my meat?
Suck my cock.
Eat my dick.
Lick my balls.
Suck my balls.
Suck my straw 'til you taste my milkshake.
I need your pussy.
I want your pussy.
Spread your legs for me.
Spread your lips for me.
Stroke my shaft with your muff.
I'm going to cream your hot little pussy.
Rock my cock in your juicy little pussy.
I'm going to fuck your hot little tail and fill you with baby juice.
Stuff me up your beautiful cunt, and hump me 'til I pass out.
Wrap your awesome legs around my ass while I fuck your sweet
    little cherry.
I want to see my juice dripping out of you.

My tongue is my strongest muscle.
I want to go muff diving.
Show me your gorgeous little cameltoe.
I want to taste your delicious pussy.
I'm going to lick and suck your sweet melons until you beg me to
    lick something else.
I'm going to lick you until you can't stand up.
Saddle up, cowgirl, and ride my moustache into the sunset.
When I get through licking your gorgeous cunt you won't be able
    to walk straight.
I'm going to hold you, and lick you, and not let you go until your
    body shakes the whole house.

Phrases for a Wife to Say

Do you like my rack?
Do you like my pussy?
Do you like my ass?
Touch me all over.
I want to feel my rack pressed against your chest.
Suck my sweet tits.
Gently suck my pussy lips.
Gently squeeze my jugs.
Want to go muff diving?
Eat my pussy.
Lick my clit.
Lick me until I beg you to stop.
Show me your meat.
I want your cock.
Pull your cock out of your pants for me.
I want to feel your shaft humping my pussy.
I need your dick inside my hot little cunt.
I want to feel your jizz drooling down my leg.
Juice me.
Fuck me.

I'm going to suck your cock dry.
Come inside me.
Cum inside me.
Ride me, cowboy.
Push your stiff meat into my hot little hole.
I'm going to fuck you until you can't stand up.
Ride my ass until your juice is dripping out my horny little
     pussy.
When I get through humping your bone, you won't be able to
     walk straight.
I'm going to spread my legs and wrap them around you until
     your cock explodes with juice inside me.

> ## A Last Word About Language:
> Many women in our family just can't think of
> things to say while having sex, whether explicit or
> naughty. If your creative side takes a vacation in
> the heat of passion, try creating **a written script**
> of whatever phrases you're comfortable with
> ahead of time, and then... yes, read it out loud
> while love-making. Sounds silly? Just try it, and
> you may be amazed at the effect!

Grandma's Ooo-aah Club

Some people have great difficulty using explicit-sexy-slang-naughty language, but nevertheless find it acceptable to listen to, and find it stimulating. If you find yourself in that boat, you can use an mp3 player with a background recording of sexual talk or just sexual moaning and groaning. One word of warning though, use headphones instead of earbuds. If you get sweaty, earbuds may give you a mild but annoying electrical shock.

And there's a major advantage to using audio recordings with headphones – you can have sex sounds as loud as you want, but no one outside your bedroom will be able to hear them!

We've been thinking about creating a web site for adults to post or download free audio files of background sex sounds of moaning and groaning, so people can find it without having to go to sites that push all sorts of extreme porn. We still haven't decided, but if we do, we'll post it at www.OooAahClub.com. If you want to weigh in with your opinion, you can let us know at www.GrandmasSexHandbook.com/feedback.htm.

Sex Tech

When we talk about sex technology, we're talking about tools and crafts with sexual applications, specifically sex toys, sex games, and tools that make remote sex possible.

Sex Toys

A sex toy can be something as common and inexpensive as a simple feather, or it can be complex and expensive, but they are all intended to enhance sexual pleasure.

You don't ever have to use one, if you don't want to, but it's okay if you do.

Sex toys can be used once in a while for a break from the routine, they may be used regularly for those who really like them, or they may be necessary for some people to compensate for specific disabilities.

As an example of the last case, one male member of Grandma's clan lost his penis in a farming accident. That didn't limit his abilities as far as cunnilingus, but his wife was one who had a strong desire for the feeling of fullness she got from vaginal intercourse. Their problem was satisfactorily resolved by the regular use of a dildo. In fact, that Grandma came to prefer the experience of her husband using a dildo on her while performing cunnilingus even more than she had previously enjoyed sex with his real penis alone.

For some men, mild erectile dysfunction may be overcome by toys like cock rings, cock vibrators, and prostate stimulators.

For some women, an orgasm can only be achieved by stimulation of the clitoris at a frequency that is easy for a vibrator, but impossible for a husband's tongue.

If you decide to try some sex toys, you don't have to spend money on them. For example, a clothes pin can work as a nipple clamp, and any kind of tool with a motor can work as a vibrator.

If you decide to keep one or more sex toys and have curious children prowling around your house, you might want to get a lock box to put them in. If they ask about the box, just tell them it's for some special things that are just for Mommy and Daddy.

So without further ado, here's a list of some common sex toys:

- Vibrators (small-bullet shaped, waterproof, variable frequencies, penis-shaped, battery-operated toothbrushes, anal, g-spot, wands, rabbits)

- Anal beads or beaded sticks
- Ball gag
- Ben Wa balls
- Body paint
- Butt plugs
- Clit suckers
- Cock rings
- Dildos
- Edible underwear
- Felt tip markers
- French ticklers
- Fucking machines
- Liquid chocolate
- Nipple clamps
- Nipple suckers
- Penis extension
- Penis sleeve
- Pocket pussies
- Sex swings
- Stimulating lubricants
- Water hose
- Temporary tattoos

> **Hot Sex Tip:** A lot of women, perhaps most, never try nipple clamps, or don't like them if they try them. But for those who do like them, get your husband to lick your nipples after they've been clamped for a minute. Wow!

Sex Games

There are board games, card games, dice, and variations on these ideas that are designed to spark romantic ideas or give you explicit sexual suggestions and fantasies. Something like, "kiss every inch of your husband from his left nipple to his manhood and back to his right nipple."

Grandma doesn't have any specific product recommendations, but you can search Amazon.com for "adult games" and find the latest ones. Amazon has both detailed descriptions and user-based product reviews.

In addition to games made with paper, cardboard, and plastic, there are many digital sex games on the Internet. Many you can play online and some you can download. Beware that some web sites have set up free sex games, online and downloadable, as a means of getting their viruses and other malware onto your computer.

Most digital games are either puzzles, adventures, or interactive cartoons, and cater to single people who want to masturbate rather than games for couples.

Remote Sex

Remote sex means you and your husband are apart, but connected by telephone or internet, and you each masturbate while you communicate and encourage each other.

The oldest form is simple telephone sex. You just talk and do your best to describe what you would normally do to and with your spouse if they were in bed with you. And you masturbate while they tell you what they would do to and with you.

The Internet adds 2 other forms of remote sex: haptics and simulations.

Haptics involve remote control of vibrators or other electronically controlled sex toys. Teledildonics refers to vibrating or thrusting dildos that use haptics. One spouse inserts a haptic toy, or straps one on, or just holds it against them, while the other spouse controls its actions from wherever else they are.

Internet simulated worlds will eventually provide "virtual sex" designed for strangers to have fantasy-assisted masturbation with each other. That will be their main market, but married couples will also be able to use them to meet each other online when they're miles apart, as a visually enhanced form of phone sex. When this technology becomes available, a husband and wife who are home together will also be able to use it to enhance their gender-reversal fantasies.

Advanced Sex Fantasies

Please read the Fantasy vs. Lust chapter before you read this topic, it's very important.

> *Grandma Caroline: I like to imagine that I'm single, have never had sex before, and that I fall so madly in love, I fall into my love's arms, and he takes me then and there. I imagine that while he's inside me for the first time, he asks me to marry him, and I say, "yes, yes, yes" as he finishes inside me.*
> *Well, that didn't happen in real life (good thing since my husband proposed in a restaurant), and I wouldn't have really wanted it to under any circumstances. Yet, I pretend it happens over and over again, so my imagination is of something immoral, but it's not real. I enjoy this fantasy a lot, but only because it's not real.*

It's okay to use your imagination while having sex.

You can pretend you're on the beach, you can pretend your spouse is a space alien, or you can pretend... anything! Our Fantasy vs. Lust chapter explains the critical difference between imagination-based fantasy and lust, and is essential to understand the full range of freedom that God gives our imaginations, and it introduces common types of sexual fantasies for Christian couples. This chapter is for those who clearly understand the principle and want to apply it to these advanced topics:

- Gender-Reversal Fantasy
- Immoral Fantasy
  - Fantasy Sanitizing Techniques
  - Adulterous Fantasy
  - Forced-Sex Fantasy
  - Group-Sex Fantasy
  - Multiple-Partner Fantasy
  - Premarital-Sex Fantasy
  - Public-Sex Fantasy
  - Same-Sex Fantasy
- Dangerous Fantasy
  - Pseudo-Bondage

Does this whole idea seem crazy to you? Well, don't feel too bad, it seems crazy to a lot of people. In our extended family, more than half of our Grandmas didn't like any of these immoral-concept fantasies. Slightly more than half of our surveyed Grandpas liked one or more. For the husbands and wives who admitted to enjoying one or more of these scenarios, they only enjoy them infrequently, just for a big change to stir up their imaginations. (sigh) Except for Grandma Rachael and her hubby... they like them all, frequently.

Gender-Reversal Fantasy

Ever wonder what sex is like for someone of the opposite sex? Well, you may not be able to find out in reality, but you can pretend to be the opposite sex and imagine what it's like.

Gender-reversal will **not** be the best sex you ever had. Then why try? Because **it can be a once-in-a-while variation that is just plain fun for both of you**. Not every sexual experience has to be an attempt to shake the Earth. And adding some adventure can help keep your romance alive, so even if a gender-reversal fantasy doesn't give you an Earth-shaking orgasm, it may help increase the intimacy and appreciation you have for each other, and *that* may lead to better orgasms at other times!

For many folks, it's difficult or impossible to be this imaginative. If you want to try, it helps a lot if your spouse also pretends to be the opposite sex at the same time. And while practice may not make perfect in this situation, it definitely makes it better. Many Grandmas who have tried this report that they had very little success when they first tried, but that after a few more times, they and their hubbies became more comfortable with the pretense, and less inhibited in their imaginations. In other words, it took repeated attempts before they really got into it.

Gender-reversal fantasy can range from simple to complex. A wife can lay on her back while her husband penetrates her and she can pretend that she's the husband with "his" wife on top. The husband can be on top of his wife but pretend that he's the wife on top of "her" husband. Or you can wear token costumes, such as the husband wearing an apron, and the wife wearing a necktie (and nothing else). On the more complex side, the wife can wear a strap-on dildo to "peg" her husband's anus. This can be fun even without trying to have orgasms. If you want to try to have orgasms while you perform a gender-reversal fantasy, the wife may need to massage her clitoris and the husband may need to manually stoke his penis.

Try it part of the time with your eyes closed, and part of the time with your eyes open. You may decide you like it better one way or the other, or that you like to alternate. Generally, the stronger your imagination, the easier it is to pretend even while your eyes are open.

You did know that you can increase your imagination by exercising it, right?

Immoral Fantasy

Sexual immorality is bad. People get hurt badly and it facilitates diseases that can cause pain, shame, and even can maim and kill. Even without the diseases, the emotional pain sexual immorality causes can be extreme.

However, there's a world of difference between sexual immorality and sexually immoral fantasy. Sexual immorality is real-world, while sexual fantasy can be imaginary only. For mentally healthy Christians couples with a healthy marriage, it is not a real-world sin to have an imagination-only sexually immoral fantasy. For a detailed explanation, *please* read the chapter on Fantasy vs. Lust, beginning on page 95.

Fantasy-Sanitizing Techniques

You can imagine absolutely anything about sex and it will not be sinful as long as it is only your imagination and not a real-life desire to have sex with someone other than your spouse. However, some folks can know this to be true and still be bothered by their conscience. Our consciences are good things, overall, but they can make mistakes.

Fortunately, for those couples who want to try immoral fantasies but whose consciences bother them, we can suggest a few ways of tweaking your imaginative scenarios to sanitize your otherwise immorally imaginative fantasies:

- Bad-Character
- Bigamy
- First-Union Cultures
- Other Worlds
- Pairing
- Pre-Gospel

Bad-Character

Instead of pretending that the real you is being sexually immoral, you can pretend that you're someone else. You can pretend that you're a prostitute, or a gold-digger, or just a sex-driven slut. Your husband can pretend he's a womanizer, a gigolo, or a selfish man who will have sex with any skirt that gives him half a chance.

The key is that you are *pretending*. It's a game while you're having sex. Once you and your hubby have orgasms and you're both coming down from your highs, you relax in each others' real-world arms, the fantasy fades away, and you warm in the knowledge that in the real world, you just had a wonderful time with your spouse, and he also had a wonderful time. You have given each other a gift of your bodies *and* your imaginations!

Bigamy

Most modern cultures don't allow a husband to have more than one wife at a time, or a wife to have more than one husband at a time, but there are some cultures that do, and it appears there always have been. Including in the Bible! In fact, the New Testament does not prohibit a man from having multiple wives, it just recommends that it's better to have only one wife. Interestingly, it doesn't address a woman having more than one husband at a time, but it's easy to argue that the lack of mention simply reflects the culture at the time, which definitely did not allow a wife to have more than one husband at a time.

Now, Grandma says if the Bible recommends only one wife per husband, we should do that in real life. However, if you're using your imagination, in your bedroom, alone with your spouse, there's no limit to what you can imagine, just for fun. If you want to pretend that your husband is one of your two husbands, that's fine. And you husband can pretend that you're wife number 7, from his harem of 27. Now, if you pretend that you're part of such a plural marriage in American society (not counting certain outlawed fringe Mormon groups), your conscience may bother you. But if you simply pretend that you're living in the Middle East 3,000 years ago, then there's no longer a social or religious restriction against your fantasy conditions.

Thus, if you can imagine a culture where an activity is legal and normal, you can modify your fantasy scenario to make your imagined world include that culture.

First-Union Culture

Some people, like Grandma Brenda, can get to a point where they understand and agree that pretending to have bad character is okay, but it still bothers their conscience to the point where they can't actually pretend that themselves. Well, a long time ago, Grandma Flora came up with this pretense that we all like a lot, including Grandma Brenda. *Especially* Grandma Brenda, because it allows her to participate in all sorts of sexual fantasies that she would otherwise not be able to.

Simply put, **we pretend that there is a culture that has marriages without weddings, and the way you get married is by having sex!** That is, having sex the *first* time, because after that, you're bound to that person and that person alone for the rest of your life. There's just one simple marriage rule: If you have sex with someone, you're married to them from then on!

You can pretend that you and your playmate (spouse) are both part of the First-Union culture, or you can pretend that just one of you is, so that one of you must explain it to the other during the fantasy. That's fun, because it creates a marriage-proposal out of any scenario that would otherwise involve pre-marital sex. And Grandma Anne, for one, likes having her husband propose many times, with each proposal followed by an hour of hot sex!

Other Worlds

You can pretend that you're on a planet other than Earth, and any type of culture and custom you want to pretend becomes the cultures and customs of your imaginary world.

Let your imagination run wild, and you may envision an Eden where the temperature is always perfect, and everyone is always naked. There are no houses, no tents, nothing to hide behind.

Or a place where people cannot communicate and develop no bonds. They just wander about and whenever they want to have sex, they just have sex with the closest person of the opposites sex that also wants to have sex, and then they go about their tasks, never to see or think about that person again.

Or you live on a world with a society that says if you have sex with someone, you must have sex with them exactly 10 times, and no more. After 10, you must move on to someone else.

Or you live on a world where the men's reproductive system has a major difference: when man has sex with a woman, he becomes chemically bonded to her unique hormone signature (like a fingerprint) and is incapable of having an erection with any other woman. Option A: When the woman starts her period, she has not become pregnant, and the man is released from the bond. Option B: If the woman becomes pregnant by the man, the man becomes her lifelong slave.

Or on your world, there are marriages, but no prohibitions against having sex with people other than your spouse because the sex drive cannot be controlled. When you get the urge, you can think of nothing else until your urge is satisfied, and that means having sex with whoever is available, regardless of marriages. Marriages are honored not for the expectation of exclusive sex, but for all the other reasons, such as emotional nurturing and financial stability.

Or... think up your own unique world – there are no limits!

Pairing

Pairing is simply pretending that the husband's and wife's roles match.

That is, if the husband wants to pretend his wife is the movie star Ann Adams, he can pretend he's Ann's husband Alan Adams. Since Alan and Ann are married to each other, you're now imagining a scenario that's doesn't include adultery.

Pairing doesn't require a husband and wife to share the same fantasy, but it can add to the illusion. While hubby is pretending he's Alan banging his wife Ann, you can pretend you're Betty, banging your husband Ben. But, if you both agree before to share your fantasy scenario, he can pretend to be Alan while you pretend to be Ann. This shared-scenario allows you both to talk in self-supporting fantasy roles: "Oh, Alan, you feel so good!" "Oh, Ann, I've loved having sex with you ever since we worked on that first movie together!"

Pre-Gospel

Imagine you're living during the first few generations of mankind. There's no Bible yet, no complex social rules, and no rigid customs regarding marriage.

You don't know what might offend other people, so you go by the laws God has written into all our hearts, treating other people the way you want to be treated. This requires you to really pay attention to other people, and sexual meltdowns may be inevitable.

Adulterous Fantasy

Okay, let's say you're reading about this, still wondering how this works. Well, if you want to *pretend* you're having sex with a real man you know other than your husband, you can use one of the sanitizing techniques described earlier, or you can pretend you're really you having sex with someone you're not married to.

There are 3 options for an adulterous fantasy: You can pretend you're married and having sex with a single man, you can pretend you're single and having sex with a man who is married to someone other than you, or you can pretend you are both married to other people.

In every scenario, your mind pretends the fantasy while you are physically having sex with your husband. Then you finish having sex, possibly after you have both had orgasms, and your fantasy thoughts fade while reality comes back into focus. The reality that you are in your husband's loving arms. Or, at least, you're laying next to your loving husband if he's passed out from physical exhaustion.

Let's say it one more time: The actual safety and security of the real world of love and trust between you and your husband gives your mind the freedom to imagine, and as your mind wanders into a dream-like fantasy, you build to a physical orgasm. As the orgasm fades, your fantasy evaporates, and you focus on reality again, still safe and secure with your husband, both of you still physically and emotionally faithful to each other alone.

Forced-Sex Fantasy

In this book, we're distinguishing forced-sex from bondage, with forced sex referring to the aggressor being overcome by an impulse, and without tying up the subject, while bondage refers to a premeditated effort to exert control over a person by using physical restraints. Sure, this distinction is thin, but there are such differences, and this is the way we chose to point them out.

So, in this book, forced-sex refers to rape by a stranger, date-rape by someone you thought was nice but turned out to be a scoundrel, or a sort-of date-rape where you and your lover have a sexual meltdown and your lover loses rational control.

In your fantasy, the aggressor can be the man or the woman. When forced-sex occurs in real-life, it's almost always the man imposing his will on the woman, but in fantasy with a husband and wife who care for each other, this fantasy is often for the wife.

How can a woman enjoy forced-sex? Because it lets her have sex with a man with bad-character without having bad character herself – she's a good person being forced, not a bad person choosing to have sex with a rogue. In fact, this is a very common fantasy for women.

A loving husband will understand that it is only the *pretense* that his wife likes, and will understand that she is 100%, absolutely, adamantly opposed to actually being forced to have sex. His role-playing must support her fantasy without going overboard.

Group-Sex Fantasy

Group sex is an orgy with men and women switching partners frequently and more than 2 people having sex at one time.

You can pretend to have group sex by pretending you are doing all that, or any of that, all the while it is only your husband in the room with you. You can enhance this kind of fantasy by you or your husband switching accents, switching costumes (or costume tokens), or using a variety of sex toys.

Multiple-Partner Fantasy

You can pretend that you're being "serviced" by one person after another, or that you are servicing one person after another. The same things that can enhance a group-sex fantasy can help this fantasy too.

Premarital-Sex Fantasy

You pretend you're engaged, are struggling to resist sexual intercourse before marriage, but become more and more intimate until one night when you're both alone in the house and... your bodies demand satisfaction with a passion that goes far beyond your rational plans of self-restraint. If you actually experienced something like this before you got married, your real-life memories may enhance this fantasy.

Public-Sex Fantasy

Here are two options for public-sex fantasies (performed in your bedroom):

Public-Sex Scenario 1: Public sex is not normal, and perhaps illegal. You and your hubby think you're completely alone in a public place, and you start having sex, only to be caught with your pants down.

Public-Sex Scenario 2: You live in a culture in which public sex is normal, and you've seen many other people doing it in every possible kind of place, but you've never done it before yourself. You're extremely self-conscious and think everyone will stop and stare at you. But you and your husband timidly start, and passerby's just keep passing by. So, you end up having sex in public for the first time, with people all around you.

Same-Sex Fantasy

Again, here are two options: You can pretend your husband is a woman and you're having woman-with-woman sex, or you can pretend you're a man and you're having man-with-man sex. Yes, this is unusual. No, this won't make you a homosexual or bisexual, just as pretending you have wings won't give you an urge to jump off the roof. Because you're *pretending*.

Dangerous Fantasy

Pseudo-Bondage

Pseudo-bondage is *playing*, can be a lot of fun, does *not* cause pain, and does *not* degrade a spouse. Examples are blindfolding and using comfortable *pretend* restraints.

An example of a pretend restraint is a long sash of cord tied to the bed frame on one end and wrapped around a wrist of the person pretending to be bound. By being wrapped, the person pretending to be bound can easily unwind the cord to get free.

Using knots around the wrists or ankles is a bad idea. If a spouse is truly bound and can't get free without assistance, what happens if the free spouse slips and falls or has a heart attack? It may be very unlikely, but it could happen. Any pretense you can have while being tied works just as well while being lightly wrapped, so just uses wraps and avoid danger.

Some couples also enjoy gags as part of a bondage fantasy. You can buy a ball-gag or other type, or use something from around the house, but if you use a household item, be *certain* that it cannot completely block the person's air flow.

Who enjoys this, and why? Well, the dominant person can be the husband or wife, and pseudo-bondage supports many master-slave type fantasies. Remember, it's *pretending*, in order to have fun.

There's another aspect worth mentioning. When a woman's ankles are tied to the bedposts so she can physically strain to close her legs but can't close them, it creates different sensations that are not possible to experience any other way. Some of the Grandmas in our family definitely like this experience *once in awhile*.

Another option on this theme is bondage-rescue. A bad person ties up the wife and the husband comes to the rescue (or vice-versa). Of course, they have sex right away to share their happiness at her being spared from whatever awful things would have happened.

Real Bondage. Real bondage is not fantasy, it's a form of masochism, inflicting real pain or degradation. Examples are using a whip and breaking the skin, or binding arms or legs into positions that stress the joints. That's a *very* bad idea. Yes, there are people who derive pleasure from giving pain and others who derive pleasure from receiving pain. Grandma says those people are broken, and their activities are not healthy.

Choking is a form of real bondage, and while the deprivation of oxygen can increase pleasure, it's extremely dangerous and has led to accidental death many times. There are many other ways to increase pleasure just as much or more, so there's no reason to risk hurting yourself or your spouse.

Play bondage: Okay when both spouses want to.
Real bondage: Never okay.

Erotic Math

Excerpts from Grandma Heather's Journal

Grandma Heather loves to crunch numbers. Even while she's having sex. None of us other Grandma's like to do that. However, after she shared some of her favorite numbers with the rest of us, we tried it out, and there were several who decided they sometimes like to think about those numbers while having sex, or whisper them to their husbands to help push them over the edge to orgasm. So just in case you might too, what kind of math does Heather find erotic? This kind:

1. How Many People Are Having Sex Right Now?

Here's Grandma Heather's favorite number: **265,306**. That's the *minimum* number of people having vaginal intercourse at the very moment you're reading this sentence.

How did she arrive at that number? In order to calculate a minimum, Heather tries to make minimum estimates. This isn't a scientific book, so we're not going to provide the numerous pages of reasoning she wrote to explain these estimates, but you may be interested in this oversimplified summary:

- Since there are well over 6 billion people in the world, she rounds down to 6 billion.
- For this calculation, Heather uses an even distribution of ages 1 to 70.
- Some people are too young to have sex, and most people wait until long after they are physically capable of sex before becoming sexually active. Heather uses a global average estimate of age 25 for becoming sexually active.
- Heather thinks the global average age at which people stop sexual activity due to death, poor health, disinterest, and all other reasons is likely to be over age 50, and Heather rounds down to 50.
- The percentage of people who can and do become sexually active is very likely to be higher, but Heather rounds this down to 80%.
- Estimates for the average frequency of vaginal sexual intercourse for sexually active people is the least reliable number, so Heather uses what she believes is a very conservative estimate of once every two weeks.

- According to some research, the average length of minutes of vaginal sexual intercourse is probably greater than five minutes, and possibly greater than 10 minutes, but Heather rounds down to 3 minutes.

Okay, those are the numbers. Here's the calculation...

Start with six billion people and keep only those between ages 25 to 50, and you have 2,228,571,428 people. Throw out the people who are not sexually active and you're down to **1,782,857,142 sexually active people** having vaginal intercourse *at least* 3 minutes every two weeks. 1,714,285,714 people times 3 minutes every 2 weeks equals 5,348,571,426 people-minutes of sex every 2 weeks. Next, there are 60 minutes per hour, 24 hours per day, and 14 days per 2 weeks, for a total of 20,160 minutes per 2 weeks. Take 5,348,571,426 people-minutes of sex per 2 weeks and divide it by 20,160 minutes per 2 weeks and you get an average of *at least* 265,306 people having sex every minute.

Every minute of every day. At least a quarter of a million people are humping right now.

For those few of you who enjoy playing around with numbers, change the estimates a little bit as see what effect it has. For example, if you estimate that when people have vaginal intercourse that they do it for at least six minutes, then the total doubles, and there are over half a million men and women copulating *all the time*.

Why does Grandma Heather like this number so much? While she's having sex, it increases her excitement to think that so many other people are having sex at the same time. As Heather says, "That's a lot of thrusting!" When we discussed this while writing this book, we all admitted that though we find it somewhat embarrassing to think about, most of us also found it to be a very stimulating thought.

Want to expand on those erotic thoughts? How about this? There are at least 265,306 people having vaginal sex all the time... while you're driving to the store, while you're shopping for groceries, while you're watching TV. Keep going... all those people are grinding pelvises into each other whenever you're taking your clothes off, every moment you're in the shower, and every time you slide into bed beside your husband. Wow, some of us find that very arousing!

2. How Many Times Do People Masturbate?

- Once per month from age 15 to age 25 is 132 times.
- Once per week from age 15 to age 25 is over 500 times.
- Once every other day from age 15 to 25 is over 1,800 times.
- Once every other day from age 15 to 65 would be over 9,000.
- Once per day from age 15 to age 65 would be over 18,000.

A person would have to average twice a day from age 12 to age 82 to hit the 50,000 mark.

3. How Much Time Do You Spend Having Sex?

34.667 hours per year based on having sex twice per week for 20 minutes per sexual episode.

If you're a sexually active husband and wife spending an average of 20 minutes having sexual intimacy during each sexual episode, including intimate foreplay, and have sex an average of twice per week, then **you spend over 34 hours per year having sex**.

The formula:
52 weeks per year * 2 times per week * 20 minutes per sexual encounter / 60 minutes per hour = 34.667 hours per year

Divide by 12 to get an average of 2.89 hours per month having sex.

Are you more active than that? Average 3 times per week and 30 minutes per sexual encounter, and you spend 78 hours per year having sex.

What's the maximum? Well, there probably aren't many people who have sex for an hour a day, every day, but if you did, you'd be spending 365 hours a year having sex, or over 30 hours per month. Grandma Heather wanted this little tidbit included in case you want a goal to shoot for!

4. How Many Men Are Licking Clits?

At least **33,920** women are having their clitorises licked as you're reading this.

If we go back to the first question, Grandma Heather estimated at least 1,782,857,142 sexually active people at any given time, and about half of those are women, so there are at least 891,428,571 sexually active women. Again, to try to derive a minimum number, we need to use very conservative estimates.

Heather hopes that most husbands lick their wives clitorises, but with no reliable measures, she estimates at least one third do. That means at least 297,142,857 women get their clits licked.

Heather also hopes that husbands who lick their wives' clits do so at least once per week, but for this equation she estimates they average at least once per month, or 12 times per year.

Finally there's the matter of how many minutes husbands average when licking their wives clitorises. Again, Grandma Heather hopes its 20 minutes or more, but to estimate a minimum as the result of the equation, we need a minimum estimate here, so Heather goes with 5 minutes.

Okay, that's the numbers for the equation, so here's the equation:

297,142,857 wives getting their clits licked for at least 5 minutes at least 12 times per year.

297,142,857 women times 5 minutes times 12 times per year equals 17,828,571,420 woman-minutes of clit-licking every year.

60 minutes per hour * 24 hours per day * 365 days per year = 525,600 minutes per year.

At least 17,828,571,420 clit-licked minutes per year / 525,600 minutes per year = at least 33,920 women having their clitorises licked every minute of every day.

5. How Many Women Are Having Orgasms?

Grandma Heather estimates that there are *at least* 1,696 women having orgasms every second of every day, including right this moment.

Once again, to try to derive a minimum number, we need to use very conservative estimates. And because women have orgasms both from sexual intercourse and from masturbation, we'll need to include both of those. We go back to the forth question to get the estimate of at least 891,428,571 sexually active women at any given time. Frequency of orgasms from female masturbation varies, but in general, sexually active women who are unmarried masturbate more often than married women, and usually have many fewer orgasms than men.

Combining both sources of orgasms for this equation, Grandma Heather estimates that the average sexually active woman has an orgasm at least once a month, though she hopes it is much higher than that.

The last estimate needed for this calculation is the average number of seconds of orgasm per orgasm. The range is from 3 to 10 seconds, so Heather estimates an average of 5 seconds.

891,428,571 sexually active women * 1 orgasm per month * 5 seconds per orgasm = 4,457,142,855 woman-seconds of orgasm per month.

4,457,142,855 woman-seconds of orgasm per month
* 12 months per year
/ 60 seconds per minute
= 891,428,571 woman-minutes of orgasm per year

60 minutes per hour * 24 hours per day * 365 days per year = 525,600 minutes per year.

891,428,571 woman-minutes of orgasm / 525,600 minutes per year = At least 1,696 women having orgasms every second of every day, including *right now*. Over one thousand, six hundred women are in the throes of erotic ecstasy while you're driving to work, while you're picking out a new pair of shoes, and while you're eating dinner. Kind of makes you want to join them, doesn't it?

6. How Many Women Are Sucking Penises?

At least 91,585 penises are being sucked by wives as you read this sentence. 24 hours a day, every day of the week, every week of the year.

Back to question 1 again, where Grandma Heather estimated at least 1,782,857,142 sexually active people at any given time. Since about half of those are men, there are about 891,428,571 sexually active men. Again, to try to derive a minimum number, we need to use very conservative estimates.

Heather hopes that most wives suck their husbands penises, but again with no reliable measures, she estimates at least one half do. That means at least 445,714,285 men get their cocks sucked by their wives.

Heather also hopes that wives who suck their husbands' cocks do so at least three times per week, but for this equation she estimates they average at least 3 times per month, or 36 times per year.

Finally there's the matter of how many minutes wives average when sucking their husbands penises. Grandma Heather estimates a minimum average of 3 minutes per occurrence.

Okay, that's the numbers for the equation, so now it's time for the equation:

445,714,285 husbands getting their penises sucked for at least 3 minutes at least 36 times per year. 445,714,285 men times 3 minutes times 36 times per year equals 48,137,142,780 man-minutes of cock-sucking every year. 60 minutes per hour * 24 hours per day * 365 days per year = 525,600 minutes per year.

At least 48,137,142,780 cock-sucking minutes per year / 525,600 minutes per year = at least 91,585 penis-sucked husbands every minute of every day.

7. How Many Men Are Having Orgasms Right Now?

Grandma Heather estimates that there are *at least* 11,024 men having orgasms every second of every day, including right this very moment.

Once again, to try to derive a minimum number, we need to use very conservative estimates. And as with women, men have orgasms both from sexual intercourse and from masturbation, so we'll need to include both of those.

We go back to question 6 to get the estimate of about 891,428,571 sexually active men at any given time. And in question 1, we estimated sexually active people are having vaginal intercourse an average of at least once every two weeks.

Frequency of orgasms from male masturbation varies. In general, sexually active men who have intercourse less often will masturbate more often, and men who have intercourse more often will masturbate less often. For this equation, based on an average of vaginal intercourse for sexually active men of only once every two weeks, Grandma Heather estimates that they compensate by masturbating at least twice in between.

Combining male orgasms from intercourse and masturbation, Heather estimates at least 3 orgasms every two weeks for sexually active men, though she suspects it is way, way higher than that.

The last estimate needed for this calculation is the average number of seconds of orgasm per orgasm. The range is from 3 to 10 seconds, so Heather estimates an average of 5 seconds.

891,428,571 sexually active men
* 1.5 orgasms per week
* 5 seconds per orgasm
= 6,685,714,282 man-seconds of orgasm per week

6,685,714,282 man-seconds of orgasm per week
* 52 weeks per year
/ 60 seconds per minute
= 5,794,285,711 man-minutes of orgasm per year

60 minutes per hour * 24 hours per day * 365 days per year = 525,600 minutes per year.

5,794,285,711 man-minutes of orgasm / 525,600 minutes per year = At least 11,024 men having orgasms every second of every day, including right now.

8. How Many Gallons Of Semen Are Being Ejaculated Each Year?

More than enough to fill 411 Olympic-sized swimming pools.

There are 16 U.S. tablespoons in 1 U.S. cup, and there are 16 cups in 1 U.S. liquid gallon.

It's estimated that the average man ejaculates 1 to 2 tablespoons of semen. If we take the low side and say the average is 1 tablespoon, then it takes 16 ejaculations to equal one U.S. cup of semen, and **256 ejaculations equals one U.S. gallon**.

891,428,571 sexually active men * 1.5 orgasms per week * 52 weeks per year = 69,531,428,538 male orgasms per year.

69,531,428,538 male orgasms per year / 160 ejaculations per gallon = at least 271,607,142 gallons of semen produced each year.

The dimensions of an Olympic pool are: 2 meters deep, 25 meters wide, and 50 meters long. A pool that size holds 660,253 U.S. liquid gallons. Of water, usually. Perhaps there has never been a swimming pool filled with semen, but all the men in the world ejaculate enough each year to fill *at least* 411 Olympic-sized swimming pools.

9. How Many Sperm Are In A Gallon Of Semen?

Over 170 billion. That's more than 25 times the population of the entire world. In *one* gallon.

The normal sperm-counts today range from 20 million per milliliter to 150 million per milliliter. For this equation, we'll use an average of 45 million per milliliter.

Just think: an average ejaculation of 15 milliliters (about 1 tablespoon) has 675,000,000 sperm. If every sperm in an ejaculation was of sufficient quality to fertilize an ovum, and if each one could be used to artificially fertilize an ovum, then it would only take 10 ejaculations to create a population of almost 7 billion people, more than all the people in the world today. Assuming of course, that you also had almost 7 billion women to carry those fertilized eggs.

Back to the gallon question: 1 U.S. liquid gallon = 3,785 milliliters; so 3,785 milliliters in a gallon times an average of 45,000,000 sperm per milliliter means that **1 gallon of semen has about 170,325,000,000 sperm.**

10. How Many Sperm Are Created Each Year?

Over 46... *quintillion.*

In question 8 we estimated at least 271,607,142 gallons of semen produced each year, and in question 9 we estimated 170,325,000,000 sperm per gallon. We just multiple those two numbers to get the minimum number of sperm per year:

That's 46,261,486,461,150,000,000 sperm.

That's at least 46 *quintillion.* Per year.

That's quite a lot of potential baby-makers!

> *These erotic-math numbers are estimates to give you something sexy to think about.*
> *No one is actually counting...*

Don't know the difference between sexual fantasy and lust?

Then you haven't read the Fantasy vs. Lust chapter, starting on page 95!

SEX FANTASY COOKBOOK

Over 100 fantasy scenarios, with over 200 "recipes", all tested and approved by Grandma Synthia.

**Submit your favorite recipe online
and win a romantic prize!**

See http://www.SexFantasyCookbook.com

Make up your own fantasy scenarios or borrow them from your favorite movies and books! The margins are wide enough for a few notes and there's some blank space at the end of this section for you to write down your own favorite recipes.

Adam & Eve

No, "Adam & Eve" isn't in alphabetical order like the rest of our recipes, but they just had to be listed first!

- *Husband = Adam; Wife = Eve:* You just woke up for the first time, in the Garden of Eden. There is a creature beside you who looks like you in many ways, but with some noticeable exceptions. He wakes up and seems surprised to see you. He moves his mouth and sounds come out. Somehow you understand what the sounds mean. Then he touches you, and you delight in the wonderful sensations. He keeps going, and you certainly don't want him to stop!

The following big-time role-reversal requires some serious imagination. Remember, you're pretending! There's no reason can't pretend you're each the opposite sex. However, gender-reversal is a little advanced, so you might want to come back to this one.

- *Husband = Eve; Wife = Adam:* You spend another day in the Garden of Eden, eating the fruit and playing with some of the animals. You lie down on the very soft, cushiony moss and fell deeply asleep. When you wake, it's morning, and there's a new creature sleeping on the ground beside you. She looks very much like you, but with a softer, rounder shape, larger breasts, and no appendage hanging between her legs. Your side is a little sore, and you feel it and notice a rib seems to be missing from that side. Somehow you realize that God has fashioned this new creature from your rib while you slept, and she is part of you, though she has a body all her own. You start touching her and she wakes up, responding with touches of her own. The touching continues and you end up laying on top and kissing passionately. That appendage between your legs feels different than it has before, and now it's big and hard and pointing away from you. It's getting in the way, but then it slips inside her. Things will never be the same again!

Abraham & Hagar

Genesis 16:1-2.
- *Husband = Abraham; Wife = Hagar:* Abraham's wife gives up on bearing children, so she has convinced him to have sex with you so that you can bear a son for him. Might as well enjoy it!

Abraham & Sarah

Genesis chapter 11:31.
- *Husband = Abraham; Wife = Sarah:* Your husband Abram turns out to be real big-shot in the Middle East. You love each other deeply and you want to bear him a child. You're disappointed that it hasn't worked yet, so you have to try over and over and over. See? There is a bright side to it!

Alien

- *Husband = alien; Wife = human female:* You've been transported into an alien space ship as a research subject. The alien has recreated a bedroom and turned himself into a human male shape based on your memories to minimize your fears. It slowly takes all your clothes off, watching your reactions very carefully. It then examines every inch of your skin with very gentle touches and strokes. Noting areas that produce greater responses, it tastes those areas by licking them.

Noting one spot produces more than the rest, it licks that spot to see how big a reaction it can cause. It then begins to probe your mouth orifice with its tongue, and probe your vagina with its penis. The appendages built into its human form seem very well suited to probing.

- *Husband = human male; Wife = alien:* You have successfully transported an Earthling into the research lab of your space ship. You use mind control to keep it docile while you unwrap the creature and touch it all over. When touching one part, it gets significantly larger. Hmm, it seems about the same size as your alien dildo, and there's no other aliens in the lab right now, so...

Archie

Remember the Archie comic books? Well, school's out and you're all alone with your heartthrob:

- *Husband = Archie; Wife = Veronica*
- *Husband = Archie; Wife = Betty*
- *Husband = Archie; Wife = Josie (& the Pussycats)*
- *Husband = Archie; Wife = Melody (a Pussycat)*
- *Husband = Archie; Wife = Val (a Pussycat)*
- *Husband = Archie; Wife = Sabrina (teenage witch)*
- *Husband = Reggie; Wife = Veronica*
- *Husband = Reggie; Wife = Betty*
- *Husband = Jughead; Wife = Ethel*
- *Husband = Moose; Wife = Midge*
- *Husband = Dilton; Wife = Betty*
- *Husband = Dilton; Wife = Miss Grundy*
- *Husband = Mr. Weatherbee; Wife = Miss Grundy*

Astronaut

- *Husband = astronaut; Wife = astronaut:* You and two men started on a 3 month voyage to the Mars colony, but since one of the guys went sleep walking outside and never came back, now it's just the two of you. And you're getting *really* tired of playing cards.
- *Husband = astronaut; Wife = astronaut:* It's just you and a guy you don't know anything about on a space mission. Past the point of no return, the heating system breaks down. Your only chance not to freeze to death is

to share body heat. Fortunately, you know how to generate lots of body heat.

Athlete

- *Husband = athlete; Wife = trainer (or reverse):* You're a world class athlete, preparing for a major competition tomorrow. A great orgasm is part of your preparation process for peak performance, and it's up to your spouse to boost your confidence with a mind-blowing experience.
- *Husband = athlete; Wife = wife:* Your husband is on a team that just won the world championship, and he scored the winning points. In the celebrations afterward, other women were fawning all over him, but you're the one he came home to, and it's time to give a very special reward like only you can.
- *Husband = husband; Wife = athlete:* Your wife has just set a new world record in her sport, and other men were practically drooling while fantasizing about how they would do what you're about to: slowly take her clothes off, caress her curves, and lick her into a state of euphoria. When she's fully satisfied with that, you put her personal scepter right where she wants it.

Bar Maid

- *Husband = customer; Wife = bar maid:* One of your favorite customers has just been dumped by his girlfriend, and he plans to get stinking drunk to dull his pain. All of sudden you realize you *really* like this guy, and the only reason you hadn't pursued him before was that you knew he already had a girlfriend. You also realize that sex prompts the brain to produce endorphins (you're a very knowledgeable bar maid), which dull pain without getting drunk. So you decide to try to pick him up on the rebound and help him create lots and lots of endorphins.
- *Husband = customer; Wife = bar maid:* Your favorite customer is the sweetest man you've ever met, and he's just landed a big promotion and come to celebrate. It turns out you're the only reason he comes to this bar, and though he's always been too shy to ask you out, the ego-boost from the promotion is enough to get him past his stage-fright. So he asks you out, you get off work and

go out to dinner where you both discover that you're perfect for each other. He takes you home, and you invite him to come inside your apartment. Then you ask him to come inside something else.

Bartender

- Husband = bartender; Wife = customer: Your fiancée dumped you and your best friend took you to a bar to help you get your mind off it. The two of you drank more than you intended to, then she got hit on and left with some strange guy, making you even more upset and lonely. You knew better, but you ordered another drink, then lost count of how many drinks you had. You wake up in the morning in a strange bed, completely naked under the covers. The bartender from the night before comes into the room, in his underwear, and sits nearby. You wonder what went on, and he explains that he tried to take you home, but your building's front door required a pin-number to get in, so he brought you to his apartment. You're naked because you threw up on your clothes, and he took them off and washed them. They're drying in the bathroom. You only half pay attention because you can't get your mind of the bulge in his shorts. You've always been a good girl, but you're getting aroused beyond anything you've ever experienced. You pull the sheet aside and though he still sits, you definitely get a rise out of him. You turn toward him and spread your legs, expecting him to take advantage, but he surprises you by starting with his tongue!

Batman/Bruce Wayne

- *Husband = Batman: Wife = woman;* You're witness a murder and are being stalked by the murder's henchmen to make sure you'll never talk. After several narrow escapes, Commissioner Gordon decides the police can't protect you well enough and he sends for the Caped Crusader. You catch glimpses of The Batman watching over you day and night. You testify, the murder and all his henchmen are sentenced to life with no parole. Case closed. Good-bye Batman. You go home, close your door, and exhale deeply for the first time since this all began. Then you're startled by a movement in your apartment. Out of the shadows emerges... your hero, The Batman, still hidden behind his mask. Neither of you speaks for a long moment, then he murmurs words of appreciation for your heroism in your steadfast determination to testify against the evil-doers. You sense his appreciation of you goes deeper than that. You slowly walk to him, then embrace him. He doesn't move. Then you kiss him, and you definitely feel him move then. You both reach up... and remove the mask between you. Then you lead him into your bedroom.

Biker

- Husband = biker; Wife = motorist: It's cold and getting dark outside when your car breaks down on a lonely road you took for the scenery and no one comes by for hours. Finally you hear someone coming – a biker who slows down and looks you over very carefully. He offers you a ride, and you debate staying with your car vs. going with him. He says this road doesn't get much traffic even in the daytime, and he'll take you to the closest phone, about 10 miles away, and you decide to go. The fact that you love his voice and he's your favorite body type has nothing to do with it. His bike doesn't have a backrest, so you have to hold on to him or fall off. You try holding on to his waist, but that feels way too insecure, so you wrap your arms around him. Without a helmet, you might die if you fall off. The wind chill makes the effective temperature drop 30 degrees at the speed he's going, and your hands are freezing. He's got gloves on, but you can't ask him for those because his hands would freeze and he wouldn't be able to drive. He seems to be thinking about the same thing, and suggests you put your hands inside his pants. You don't. For awhile. Then you really don't have a choice, so you worm them in, and oops, either he's not wearing undershorts or you burrowed too deep – your hands are too cold to tell. You try to keep your hands as still as possible and wait for the nightmare to end. Then the road gets bumpy, very bumpy, and while your hands are gripping each other they're also bouncing up and down on him. He finally gets you to the motel, and get off, and you realize he's colder than you are, having taken the brunt of the cold air. And bad news, the motel's phone lines are down! Worse news, your purse is gone, somewhere in the middle of the road miles away, apparently. The biker has just enough cash for one room with a double bed. There's no discussion because there seem to be no other options: he takes the room and you both go in and turn the heater on full blast. You take turns taking hot showers and then go to bed both fully dressed and with an agreement not to touch each other. All night long you dream about that ride, and what had been a nightmare turns into an erotic dream. When you wake up, you're embarrassed to find yourself with your arm over him, and he was already awake. Before you have time to think, he turns toward you and kisses you. Your brain now has no chance, your body takes over and it's your turn to give the biker a ride.

Boss

- *Husband = employee; Wife = boss (wear a skirt and panties):* You're the boss in your office, and you haven't had sex since your husband died two years ago. Your libido was dormant until recently, when you started fantasizing about a new employee. Then one day you learn that he's a widower, and it just so happens that the two of you need to work late together. Alone. When you get through with the work and start filing the papers away, you use a ladder to put a box up on a shelf and he uses a filing cabinet right next to you. Your foot slips and he turns to catch you, putting his face right into your crotch. You freeze for a moment, wondering how to react. Then, to your surprise, he inhales, deeply, and moans. He doesn't move. You start to wrestle loose and tell him to let you go, but you hear yourself saying, "Eat me." Your reservations evaporate into ecstasy as he lifts your skirt, pulls your panties aside and begins to lick your clit.
- *Husband = boss; Wife = employee:* You've been job hunting for weeks, but have found nothing. You have no family still alive, no close friends, make very little money, you live alone and frugally, but you're starting to lose ground financially. One day your boss tells you he needs you to work late, which is strange, because there's really not much work you can do after hours. You knock on his door at 5:30, to find out what he wants you to do. He tells you to come in, then gets behind you and locks the door. He comes straight to his

point. You make him horny, and he wants you to fix the problem you created. You try to leave, and he makes it clear – if you don't satisfy him, he'll find an excuse to fire you. You're no stranger to sex, but you don't want to be forced. Still, when he starts undressing you, you don't fight. You decide you'll let him do whatever he wants and start trying even harder to find another job. When you see his package, you feel desire, and you chastise yourself for it, but you can't help but enjoy the physical aspect of it.

- *Husband = boss; Wife = employee:* 5:30, time for everyone but you and the boss to go home. 5:45, time to go into your boss's office, lock the door and hike up your skirt or whatever he wants. If he wants to get you off first, you'll be there until 6:30, otherwise, you'll be able to leave by 6:00.

Options: *Boss is single, Boss is married, employee is single, employee is married.*

- *Husband = boss; Wife = employee:* You notice your boss often works late alone. After meeting his Mrs., you suspect you know why. She seems like a classic sophisticated socialite who would effectively manage a household staff and spend her time scheduling fancy dinner parties, but might be an iceberg in the bedroom. You decide to see how appreciative your boss might be to a seductive woman. It might not guarantee a promotion or raise, but putting out in order to move up is a career plan you're comfortable with.

Builder

- *Husband = builder; wife = homeowner;* While at work, you notice a man working across the street, building a small new office building, then you find yourself glancing out the window far more often than usual. You also start fantasizing about Mr. Builder. And that's before the day he takes his shirt off while unloading his truck. Wow. The next day his truck is parked outside while you're coming in from lunch, you notice the side of his truck says "no job too small", and you impulsively get his attention to ask about adding a deck to your house. He gets your address and promises to come over that evening to give you an estimate. While waiting, you put on your favorite perfume. He comes, looks things over, and gives you an estimate. You snuggle up to him and ask him if there's *anything* you can do to get a discount. He seems caught off guard, so you follow up by starting to unbutton his shirt, and that gets him started. You slowly undress each other, and you expect to end up on your couch in short order, but instead he holds you by the waist and lifts you straight up, as if you weighed nothing. You wrap your legs around his waist and he ever so slowly lowers you onto himself. You move up and down as he groans, and you wonder how long it will be before he has to lay down, but he stands like a pillar. When he's close, you put your tongue in his ear, and he explodes inside you, to your amazement, still standing. You tell him you don't really want a deck, but you want him to come back again for dinner. He says he's been wanting to eat something since he first met you, and now he can't wait.

Butterflies

- *Husband = monarch butterfly; Wife = nymphalidae butterfly;* You and your lover enjoy life and each other as you mate in the air, flying through the fields and forests.

Casanova

- *Husband = Casanova; Wife = house guest;* You've heard of the legendary womanizing of Casanova, and are concerned that the group traveling in your carriage agree to stop at his estate overnight. At dinner, he lavishes his attentions on all the women in attendance, including his wife. You're relieved that she is at home to prevent him from nocturnal wanderings. That night, however, you are aroused to be sleeping in a bed you know to belongs to him. You finally get to sleep dreaming of what it might be like to feel him inside you, slowly moving up and down, then down, down, until his mouth is on your flower, and his tongue is caressing you, and slowly, slowly, you realize you are no longer dreaming. You may scream, but it won't be for help.

Casper and Wendy

- *Husband = Casper the friendly ghost; Wife = Wendy the good little witch;* You're being raised by your 3 evil aunts and your best friend – your only friend – is

Casper, who is being raised by his 3 evil uncles. You're both finally old enough to get married, and this is your wedding night. You've never used your magic for anything but good, much to your aunts' dismay, and now you use your magic to give Casper enough physical presence to caress you and penetrate you. And that is definitely good.

Castaways

- *Husband = pilot; Wife = passenger:* After you're unjustly fired, you decided to take a real vacation before starting the job hunt again. A special deal included a chartered flight on a sea plane to an isolated island in the Bahamas. After landing you at your destination, the pilot discovers the battery in his plane has gone dead. The engine can't start, and the radio won't work. Your parents died a few years ago and you have no other relatives, so no one is going to come looking for you. Mr. Pilot says he filed a flight plan, but he suspects no one at the tiny airstrip on the coast of Georgia will ever check it. When your bottled water runs out, the island has a groundwater pool that may keep you alive, but you only brought enough food to last you for 2 weeks. That means only a week with 2 people, so you both spend your days trying to learn how to spear fish, weave a fishing net, find edible vegetation. At night you sleep on the bed in the only cottage on the island, and he sleeps on the floor. He never complains, but you can tell it's very uncomfortable. After two months you've gotten to know each other very well, you like each other, and you have no real prospects for rescue. You've been thinking more and more about sharing your bed. If you do, how are you going to explain that you had a doctor put in an IUD the year before, but still convince him that you never really needed it?

Remember the TV show Gilligan's Island?
- *Husband = Gilligan; Wife = Ginger*
- *Husband = Gilligan; Wife = Mary Ann*
- *Husband = Gilligan; Wife = Mrs. Howell*
- *Husband = The Professor; Wife = Ginger*
- *Husband = The Professor; Wife = Mary Ann*
- *Husband = The Professor; Wife =Mrs. Howell*
- *Husband = The Skipper; Wife = Ginger*

- *Husband = The Skipper; Wife = Mary Ann*
- *Husband = The Skipper; Wife = Mrs. Howell*
- *Husband = Mr. Howell; Wife = Mrs. Howell*
- *Husband = Mr. Howell; Wife = Ginger*
- *Husband = Mr. Howell; Wife = Mary Ann*
- *Husband = headhunter; Wife = Ginger*
- *Husband = headhunter; Wife = Mary Ann*
- *Husband = headhunter; Wife = Mrs. Howell*

Remember the movie Castaway, starring Tom Hanks?

- *Husband = castaway; Wife = Wilson*

Carpenter

- *Husband = carpenter; Wife = apprentice:* You get a job as a novice carpenter working under the tutelage of the man whom you later marry. Occasionally on remodeling jobs, when no one else is around, you both test the owners' bed in the master suite. You find that kinky enough that you start carrying a special bag with towels so you can't make too big a mess, and you sometimes take on contracts just because you hope to get into someone else's bedroom.

Cat Woman

- *Husband = man: Wife = Cat Woman;* Rowr! You're the sexy object of desire of every virile man, and you know how to tease... without going too far... except with this one guy, who really makes you *purrrrr!*

Cheerleader

- *Husband = cheerleader; Wife = cheerleader;* At your college, male and female cheerleaders team up, and you *really* like your partner. And you *really* like the lifts and catches that require him to put his hand on your crotch. Judging from the bulge he gets when working with you, he likes it, too. You decide to get him to practice with you at your house.
- *Husband = jock; Wife = cheerleader;* There are lots of jocks, and most are empty-headed, but you really like one guy who's not only buff, he has a great sense of humor that indicates an actual working mind. Hello's graduate to short greetings, and then to short conversations, and it's obvious that he appreciates your

mind. You invite him home after school, when no one else is around, and decide to find out how much he likes your famously stacked body.

- *Husband = geek; Wife = cheerleader;* You've been a cheerleader since elementary school and have always been around athletes. But in high school, when you get asked out by geek, you accept as a mercy date. Much to your surprise, he's thoughtful, considerate, and very interesting. You go on another date, and then another, and another. It finally dawns on you that you *really* like this guy, and you decide you could not do better than to plan your future together with him. You plan to get him alone at your home after school to give him your virginity, and are *very* pleasantly surprised to discover that he has a very muscular tongue.

Chemical Warfare Researcher

- *Husband = researcher; Wife = researcher:* You work in a chemical research laboratory trying to create a nerve gas with only a psychological effect that will render soldiers incapable of fighting by increasing their sex drives to extreme levels. You and your male colleague have had great success, judging from your animal tests, but then you have a terrible accident: the gas leaks into your office!

Cleopatra & Mark Antony

- *Husband = Marcus Antonius; Wife = Queen Cleopatra:* You're the Queen of Egypt, and you can't just fool around with any commoner. Good thing for you that Mark Antony is on your social level and completely captivated by your charms.

Clothing Maker

- *Husband = clothier; Wife = customer;* You order a new made-to-fit swimsuit, and the male clothier has to measure you for the fitting. Several times. Once it's finished and you try it on, he has to pull it and primp it to make sure it fits well, especially in the crotch and around the breasts, where he has to carefully check to determine how much fabric to add or take away. You decide to order another custom swimsuit, and then another. He finally gets the hint and starts checking for fit without any cloth at all.

- *Husband = customer; Wife = clothier;* Your customer purchases underpants from you, and you have to alter them to fit. Of course, you have to smooth out any wrinkles before you can plan the alterations. And there are lots of wrinkles. Then you have to decide whether to alter the size for before or after his appendage is inflated.

Clothing Inspector

- *Spouse = inspector; Spouse= citizen;* You have to randomly check people's clothes, and particularly their underwear, while they're wearing them, to ensure their fit complies with government standards. The way you do the job, you earn more money from tips than wages.

Comatose Patient

- *Husband = patient; Wife = nurse;* You're the newly assigned midnight-shift nurse in a ward of comatose patients. The only real tasks are to monitor and give sponge baths, since even comatose patients still sweat a little bit, and because of the light load, you're the only one on duty. While most nurses would skimp when bathing a comatose patient, you're as thorough as always, which leads you to discover one male patient with an unique reaction for a man in a coma – he gets an erection when you bathe his penis, and it happens every time. The phenomena causes you to think about it more and more, until it begins to become an obsession, and an erotic one at that. Finally, you come to work with a secret in your purse, a condom, and you can hardly wait until the second shift leaves so you can test your theory. And it works: with a little stroking to get him hard, he is a living, breathing dildo, and you make the most of it.
- *Husband = orderly; Wife = patient;* You're a comatose patient in a ward with a newly assigned midnight-shift orderly. Although you cannot move or control your body at all, you have some consciousness and can sometimes sense your body. The orderly's only real tasks are to monitor and give sponge baths, and because of the light load, he's the only one on duty. Out of all the patients,

he is enthralled with your beauty. One night his desire for you takes over and he has sex with your unresponsive body. The next night, he takes advantage again, but this time he spends a few minutes licking your clitoris before penetrating you. Night after night, he continues this routine, and over weeks, it has an impact: you begin to sense your body more and more. Eventually, it reaches a point of awareness of what is happening to you, and then it becomes the focus of your consciousness. And eventually, your body starts to respond physically, imperceptibly at first, but finally your orderly notices an ever so tiny reaction as he licks you. Stunned, and excited at the prospect of bringing you out of your lost world, he spends more and more time each night performing cunnilingus, and ever so slowly, your body reacts more and more. Eventually, you moan, and a week later you have an orgasm. Two weeks after that, your orderly is devotedly licking you again and your eyes open for the first time in no telling how long. You look around and see that you're in a hospital, you know you're mind has been in a lost world for a very long time. You know there is a man licking between your legs, and you know he is the reason you have awoken. You build to an unavoidable climax, and to his joy, you speak for the first time in years. And your first words are to beg him to come inside you.

Competitor

In the future, there are devices that can monitor brain waves and tell if a man or woman is having an orgasm or faking. And it can determine the strength and duration of orgasms. Initially for research purposes, the devices are made to record all orgasms in a computer system. Then some researchers start competing to see who can give their spouses the most, strongest, and/or longest orgasms.

- *Husband = researcher; Wife = wife:* You poor girl, your husband is determined to inflict you with orgasm after orgasm to win an office bet.
- *Husband = husband; Wife = researcher:* You've been more successful than most of your colleagues in getting your husband to have orgasms, and now it's the final week of a big bet and you have just one competitor who's barely ahead of you. If you can catch up and pass

her, you'll win a big shopping trip! If only your husband can keep it up...

Con Artist

- *Husband = con man: Wife = mark;* The man you were sharing your bed with turns out to be a man who can convince almost anyone about almost anything. He pretended to be a rich and well respected business man, falling in love with your in order to set you up to steal your money. You told him you learned the truth and threw him out. He did leave, but now he's back, risking arrest in order to... propose marriage, insist on a prenuptial agreement that gives him nothing, promise to get a real job, and whatever else it takes to get you to spend the rest of your life with him. Which is exactly what you planned from the beginning.

Concubines and Absalom

King David's son Absalom rebelled against David's rulership and had sex with David's concubine in front of a large crowd to make the breach irreconcilable. "So they pitched a tent for Absalom on the roof, and he lay with his father's concubines in the sight of all Israel." 2nd Samuel 16:20-22

- *Husband = Absalom; Wife = concubine;* Absalom goes into the tent, and you're brought in to him. Thousands of people are watching you go in, knowing you're going to have sex with the King's son and usurper, and when you come out, they'll still be there watching, knowing you just had sex. You wonder how many of the women watching wish they were in your shoes?

Cop

- *Husband = cop; Wife = resident;* A cop shows up at your door and explains that there's a drug dealer living across the street. You agree to cooperate by letting them use your bedroom to spy on the drug dealer. During the long night hours, you get more and more chummy with the cop. When the dealer leaves for awhile, the cop has some time to spare, and you want him to demonstrate his handcuffs on you.
- *Husband = thief; wife = cop;* You're the lone responder to an alarm at a sex toy store, and you catch the thief leaving with his arms full of products. He's a good

looking guy and you make him put them all back, then make sure the store's locked before you leave. You tell dispatch it was a false alarm and you're going to take your lunch break at home. You don't tell them it will be with a guy in handcuffs.

- *Husband = cop; wife = speeding driver;* You get pulled over by a great looking cop. In fact ,he's the same great looking cop who pulled you over a week ago at the same place. And you've been speeding here ever since, hoping to see the same guy again. This time you want a lot more than a ticket, which is fine with him.
- *Husband = cop; wife = citizen;* You called the police to report a crime but refused to tell the operator what it was. An officer shows up at your door, and you explain that the crime is that you've been wanting to have sex for months, but you haven't been able to find a guy who likes to eat pussy. Fortunately for you, this cop is no vegetarian when it comes to sex.
- *Husband = citizen; wife = cop;* The whole town is talking about how the town council is railroading through a set of regulations everyone hates, and how one man was arrested for disorderly conduct for refusing to stop objecting during a meeting. You're giving him a ride home after he posted bail, and you're impressed that he risked jail to stand up for his principles when no one else would. You're also impressed that he's single and he invites you into his apartment for coffee.

Cowboy / Cowgirl

- *Husband = cowboy; Wife = cowgirl:* You're daughter of the ranch owner and you're good at every job on the ranch. A great-natured, good-looking young man came to work for your father a few years before, and has just been promoted to ranch foreman. You decide he's just the man to become co-owner with you someday, and your marriage is announced with joy all around. Waiting for marriage, though, turns out to be a lot harder than you expected.
- *Husband = cowboy; Wife = traveler:* Your car breaks down on a lonely country road with no cell phone towers in range. You have no choice but to start walking, and it starts getting dark. A man comes riding

up on a horse in the field next to the road and offers to put you up for the night and take you to town in the morning. It seems like the best course of action, and you discover he's a complete gentleman as well as the owner of a large ranch. Without air conditioning to make noise, you have trouble sleeping and you look out the window when you hear a screen door open and close. You see your cowboy rescuer going to a late night swim in the back yard. You decide to join him. He doesn't mind that you don't have a swimsuit.

- *Husband = historian; Wife = cowgirl:* You inherited the ranch you grew up when your father died a few years back, and although you can manage the ranch very well, you've been very lonely, and there are very few eligible men that you have opportunity to contact. One evening you get a phone call from a historian who wants to interview you about your father's experiences in Viet Nam, and you agree. It turns out he knows more about your father's experience than you did, but a common appreciation of your father is just the kindling to build a roaring fire of a romance.

Damsel

- *Husband = ruffian; Wife = damsel:* You are a lady-in-waiting sent on an errand through the woods, and it's dusk as you make your way home and you're accosted by a thief. You have no money, but he's happy to take another form of treasure. After all, that's why you took this path. Again.

David & Bathsheba

- *Husband = King David; Wife = Bathsheba:* You took a luxurious bath on the roof patio of your house next to the King's wing of the Palace, knowing you could be seen from his chambers, and you weren't surprised to be summoned to him. The King looks as good close up as he did from a distance, and you intend to find out what he looks like all over.

Doctor

- *Husband = gynecologist; Wife = patient;* You're single, your doctor's single, and you think he's more than professionally interested by the way he's gotten flustered and apologetic. Now, how can you get him to help you satisfy your libido?

- *Husband = patient; Wife = urologist;* Your patient is your favorite, being great looking and having a great outlook on life despite his wife dying the year before. He's in because he's been having increasing difficulty, and it sounds like he may be getting an enlarged prostate. You put on a glove to perform a digital rectal exam, using your finger in his anus to feel the prostate gland through the wall of his rectum. You ask him to lower his pants and shorts, and most guys turn around first and lower their pants just enough, but this guy drops them to the floor before turning around, and you're very favorably impressed. While you're feeling his prostate, he gets an erection, for which he apologizes, and you tell him not to worry about it. You tell him his prostate does feel enlarged as you throw the glove away, but not to pull up his pants so you can check his testicles for lumps while they're "handy". While you do that, he involuntarily moans, for which he apologizes. You decide to ask him to dinner, and you decide before he pulls his pants up, you're going to give him a compelling reason to say yes.
- Husband = medical student; Wife = medical student; Studying from a book is one thing, learning terminology is easy, knowing first-hand how the organs of the opposite sex work is something else altogether, so you and your fellow student decide to explore each other, just for academic purposes, of course.

Dogs

- *Husband = dog: Wife = dog;* You're a happy dog, well cared for and without a worry. Whenever you get in heat, you just put your rear end where a male dog can satisfy your itch.

Drill Instructor

- *Husband = Drill Instructor: Wife = recruit;* You've just started Sex Boot Camp, and you have to do whatever the loud, demanding DI tells you to do.
- *Husband = recruit: Wife = Drill Instructor;* You're the DI for a new Sex Boot Camp trainee. It's your job to turn this novice into a sex expert, whether they like it or not.

Elephano

- *Husband = elephano; Wife = woman;* You're in bed with a creature that has a flexible nose several feet long and just the right width to... satisfy your intimate desires.

Erotic Models

- *Husband = model; Wife = model:* Artistic painters need human models, and painters of erotic art need human models performing sex. You and your husband perform sex acts while the students in the painting class watch.

Evil Test Subjects

- *Husband = test subject; Wife = test subject:* Bad guys have locked you and some strange man into a room and won't let you out until you put on a sex show they find satisfactory. They have cameras mounted in the ceiling and walls, and apparently plan to have customers watching over the internet. Neither one of you have any intention of giving in to their evil demands, but then the room temperature goes up. Eventually you both strip down to your underwear due to the extreme heat, but remain committed to no contact. Then they start piping some kind of gas into the room, and both of your sex drives get stronger and stronger. It gets to the point where all you can think about is the other's almost naked body, their beautiful, sensual, erotic body. Finally there's a touch – just one little touch, and your passions explode in a fiery frenzy, oblivious to everything else.

Fairy

- *Husband = man: Wife = fairy;* You're a fairy, able to grant wishes to mortals when you wish. Your attention becomes fixed on one guy, and you decide to reveal yourself to him and offer him a wish. To your delight, he wishes you to share his bed.

Fashion Model

- *Husband = designer; Wife = fashion model;* The designer is having an after-party at his house, you think it's a good career move to get him alone in his bedroom.

Fashion Show Assistant

- *Husband = changing assistant; Wife = fashion model;* The cute replacement their hired at the last moment before the fashion show is very good at helping you get out of one outfit and into the next. You seem hypersensitive to his touch, and you feel highly erotic as you strut on the runway, having your best show ever, and being offered a fat new contract when the show's over. You find the assistant before he gets away, because you want to keep him close from now on. Very close.

Firefighter

- *Husband = fire-fighter; Wife = civilian;* The apartment next door catches fire and spreads to your apartment. You pass out from smoke and wake up being carried by a fire-fighter. He puts an oxygen mask on you to help you recover and he chats to help you calm down. When he learns you have no friends or family in town, and you purse just went up in flames, he offers to let you stay at his house. Which won't be an imposition for him since he's single and available.

First-Time Lover

- *Husband = groom; Wife = bride;* You've never been naked in front of a man and you really hope he likes your body. And you wonder what it's going to be like to feel another person inside your body.

Fitness Buff

- *Husband = fitness buff; Wife = fitness buff;* Sometimes you wake in the middle of the night and have trouble getting back to sleep. You discover that the best thing to do is go to your apartment building's fitness center and getting a workout. After some exercise and a shower, you can get right back to sleep and even feel well rested the next morning. In fact you develop a fondness for that quiet time alone in the sauna, pool, hot tub, or on the exercise equipment. One night you stay in the hot tub a little too long and get dizzy. You get out and go to the changing room showers, only to walk right into a naked man face-to-uh, face. You get frightened and start hitting him in self-defense, but it eventually dawns on you that he's not attacking, just trying to ward off your blows. Then it dawns on you that the room doesn't look quite right. Then it dawns on you that you're in the men's locker room. You know you need to start apologizing, but your mind focuses on the fact that while he was defending himself, he was too busy to cover up, and there was a *lot* to cover up. And he's still standing there naked in case you start hitting him again. Impulsively, you start to offer him your towel, which just makes you appear even more crazy. So, that's how you met this guy. Surprisingly, he was understanding, and over time, you two became occasional midnight workout partners. Tonight you decide to see if you can get him to come to your apartment for a workout.

Foreigner

- *Husband = neighbor; Wife = neighbor;* You're both single and available, but you speak different languages.

Fred Flintstone

- *Husband = Fred; Wife = Wilma;* Fred's on his way home and you want to get pregnant. You want to have a girl and name her "Pebbles", but first you have to get Fred to rock your world in bed.

Fuck-Buddy

- *Husband = fuck-buddy; Wife = fuck-buddy;* One of you needs sex, the other gives it to them. Quick or slow. No hassles.

Furniture Salesperson

- *Husband = furniture salesman; Wife = wife;* You visit your husband at his furniture sales job during lunch hour and sneak away to a remote bed display to have sex, hoping you don't get caught by his boss, co-workers, or customers.
- *Husband = furniture salesman; Wife = customer;* You wander into a furniture store, lie down to test a mattress in an enclosed showcase room, and accidentally fall asleep. You have a very erotic dream that wakes you up, and you can tell by the lights and silence that the store is closed. You find the situation highly arousing and have no sense of fear or concern, so you decide that before you start trying to find a way out, you'll enjoy the

privacy and play with yourself. Then you're discovered by a salesman who was working late on paperwork and heard your moans. He offers to help you out.

Gardener

- *Husband = gardener; Wife = homeowner;* Your husband is out of the country on business again, but your hormones aren't taking a vacation. Your gardener seems more than qualified to tend to your needs.

Genius

- *Husband = genius; Wife = neighbor;* You learn that your new neighbor is single and available, but hear that he's "quirky". You decide to find out for yourself, and discover that his social skills are undeveloped, but he's a genius physicist with a strong and sophisticated sense of humor. You become good friends and like to watch movies together on Saturday nights. After one movie, he simply asks you for sex. You simply take him into the bedroom and start taking his clothes off. And you simply have a wonderful time.
- *Husband = handler; Wife = genius;* You're a genius working as an elite problem solver for a company that provides a handler to act as your assistant and meet your every need so that you can focus exclusively on each assignment. He's particularly good at keeping your libido satisfied.

Ghost

- *Husband = ghost; Wife = widow;* After your husband dies, you can almost still feel him at night in bed. No, you *can* still feel him. As long as the lights are off, you can feel his entire body, and even his breath. And he still likes to do the same things he used to do.

Option: reverse roles.

Goldilocks

- *Husband = Bear; Wife = Goldilocks;* You got lost in the woods early hours ago, now you're hungry and tired. You come upon a cottage and knock at the door, but there's no answer. Too tired to go elsewhere, you try the door and it is unlocked. You help yourself to some food and then collapse onto the bed and fall fast asleep. You awake with a start to realize that someone is sitting on the bed next to you. Your eyes come into focus, and to your terror, it is a man-sized bear, but before you have time to faint, it speaks! At first it's words are reassuring, and you think it won't eat you. But then it demands payment for the food, and it eats you after all, all night long.

Good Citizen

- *Husband = citizen; Wife = citizen;* This is "Random New World", a take-off based on Alexander Huxley's book (shocking when it was first published) "Brave New World", where society is controlled by professional planners. In this version, the planners send a signal for adults to have sex, and you must have sex with whichever member of the opposite sex is closest. So, wherever you and your husband are when you want to have sex, pretend you don't know each other and the signal has just gone off. You're now required by law to get each other off.

Greek god / goddess

- *Husband = god; Wife = mortal;* A god has come down from Olympus looking for some entertainment. If you can get him under your skirt, he'll probably make sure you're well taken care of from then on.
- *Husband = mortal; Wife = goddess;* You come down from Olympus to see what the mortals are doing and take special interest in a cute guy. He seems resistant to your charms, but you can be very persuasive.
- *Husband = god; Wife = goddess;* You and a god bet each other as to who can give the other an orgasm first. Whoever loses has to be the other's love slave for a week.

Gunslinger

- *Husband = gunslinger; Wife = saloon girl;* You like a local gunfighter, and when a stranger comes to challenge him, you decide to keep him from finding out by keeping him in your bedroom until the stranger leaves town.

Gymnast

- *Husband = fan; Wife = gymnast;* You're a world-class gymnast, and you have a big fan who makes no apologies for ogling your crotch at every opportunity. After winning a big competition, you want to give him a better view in a very private celebration.

Hero / Heroine

- *Husband = hero; Wife = fiancée;* The love of your life has just come with news that he's been called to war and must leave in the morning, perhaps never to return. There is no one available to perform an emergency wedding, but you don't care. You just finished your period, with only a few spots all day, so it's unlikely that you could get pregnant, and you're willing to risk it to be intimate with him at least once.
- *Husband = fiancée; Wife = heroine;* Your wedding was only a few weeks away, but word has come that an invading army is close at hand. As one of the best archers in the land, you must leave within hours, and your fiancée, with a hand crippled in the last war, must stay and supervise the defense of your village. He comes to your cottage to say a quick and intense goodbye, and you cannot resist spending a few minutes in bed, perhaps for the only time before you die in battle.

Honeymooners

- Husband = newlywed; Wife = newlywed: This is your wedding night, and neither of you knows anything about sex. You'll just have to try to figure how things work and make the best of it.

Household Slave

- *Husband = owner; Wife = slave;* The plantation owner has always give you special consideration, and you have always admired him. One night after his wife dies, he wants more from you than your normal duties.
- *Husband = slave; Wife = owner;* Your houseboy has always been perfectly obedient. One afternoon months after you received news that your husband was killed in

the war, your hormones take control and you find out just how obedient he is.

Human Sex Pet

There are two sub-species of humans: the Thinkers have normal reasoning skills like all real humans; the Pets have no critical thinking skills. Thinkers own, feed, and care for their Pets. Pets just eat and sleep. However, if well trained, they can use toilets, brush their own teeth, and most importantly, perform any sexual activity you want them to. And you may need to use a leash while you're training them. And you need to keep their sex drives satiated to keep them from humping the neighbors' pets.

- *Husband = sex pet; Wife = thinker;* You really love your sex pet, and it seems like his tongue could go on forever. What other tricks can you teach it?
- *Husband = thinker; Wife = sex pet;* You really love your owner, and it seems like he really likes you to do things with that short-stick thing between his legs. You live to make him happy, if only you can understand what he wants you to do. And you really like the way he rewards you, too.

Hypnotist

No, hypnotism doesn't allow someone to make you do something you wouldn't normally do. But because you're pretending, it can do that and more!

- *Husband = hypnotist; Wife = subject:* You volunteer to be hypnotized as part of a stage show in Las Vegas. It all appears normal as far as the audience knows, but before the hypnotist appears to bring you out of the trance, he whispers into your ear. That night, without thinking, you rise and go to his room.
- *Husband = subject; Wife = hypnotist:* You ask for volunteers to be hypnotized as part of your Las Vegas act, and tonight you have many volunteers to choose from. Ah, you pick the man you spotted when he first entered the room – how you hoped he would raise his hand, and now you plan on getting him to raise something else. You put him through a fake-awakening so everyone thinks he's back to normal, but that night when you knock at his door, a set of commands you whispered earlier take control of him.

Indiana Jones

- *Husband = Jones; Wife = former best friend:* Jones whirls into town on another adventure, and needs your help. Before you help him with what he needs, you demand his help between your legs.

Isaac & Rebekah

Genesis 24

- *Husband = Isaac; Wife = Rebekah:* It's your wedding day. And you've never met your husband before. The festivities keep you apart except for few moments and the ceremony, but now it's time for your first night together.

Jacob & Leah

- *Husband = Jacob; Wife = Leah:* It's your wedding night. Jacob has served your father for seven years on a pledge that he will marry your younger sister Rachael, but since it is the custom for the eldest daughters to be married first, you father has substituted you in the wedding, covered by veils. Now as you wait for him, you must continue the ruse until after he has consummated the marriage.

Jacob & Rachael

- *Husband = Jacob; Wife = Rachael:* Jacob served your father for 7 years on a pledge that he would marry you, but your father tricked him by hiding you and sending your older sister in your place. Jacob was angry when he found out, because he loves you, but your father made him a deal that he could still marry you if he worked another 7 years, and Jacob agree. Now it's finally your wedding night. This time Jacob insists that you make love for the first time with your face uncovered.

Jailer

- *Husband = jailer; Wife = prisoner:* The other women in jail dislike you and mean to harm you if they can. You've been okay so far because the jailer who assigns cells has kept you in a cell by yourself, so he can spend time alone with you.

- *Husband = prisoner; Wife = jailer:* You're responsible for picking prisoners to be "trustees" who get to be out of their cells a lot in exchange for doing chores. You have one prisoner that you want for a very special chore in the bed of a spare cell.

James Bond

- *Husband = James Bond; Wife = love interest;* You attend an elegant dinner party alone to make new business contacts, and you're attracted to a charming cad who's only interested in one thing.

Judah & Tamar

Don't remember these two? Bet you will after you act out this fantasy a time or two. Genesis 38.

- *Husband = Judah; Wife = Tamar:*, Judah is obligated to have his only remaining son marry you, but he refuses to do so. You hear that he is making a trip, so you cover yourself with veils like a prostitute and wait by the road. Your trick works, and when he passes by, he wants to hire you, without knowing who you really are.

King

- *Husband = king; Wife = citizen:* The King is bored with all his wives and wants someone new to share his bed tonight. His servants pick you out at the market, and you have no choice but to comply. You decide to make the most of the situation and see if you can keep the King from ever getting bored with you.

King Solomon & Queen of Sheba

- *Husband = Solomon: Wife = Queen of Sheba;* Invited to meet the world's most famous king, known for both his wisdom and his wealth, you bring an entourage intended to impress. But it is not your entourage that captures the King's attention, but your beauty. Will you share the bed of the King of Israel and forever link your kingdoms?

Knight

- *Husband = knight; Wife = lady:* A boy you grew up with was your best friend until he was taken away from your village to serve as a squire to a royal Knight. He became a Knight himself, was granted an estate, and has come to take you with him as his bride.

Lifeguard

- *Husband = lifeguard; Wife = swimmer:* You get too far out from the beach, can't make it all the way back, and start to drown. The next thing you know, you're on the beach, and an incredible guy has been giving you mouth-to-mouth resuscitation. His mouth is still inches from yours, in case he need to give you any more air. He introduces himself and you offer to take him home to thank him all night long.
- *Husband = lifeguard; Wife = swimmer:* Darkness is falling rapidly as the last of the beachgoers leaves and the great looking lifeguard you've been flirting with all day finally starts down from his tower. You run over and snatch his towel and he gives chase. He catches up to you in the surf, and you trip on the towel. You turn as you fall, and he falls on top of you, straddling your waist. As he kisses you, you can feel his hardness pressed against you, and you don't object as he removes your swimsuit.

Lion

- *Husband = lion; Wife = woman;* You are alone in the Savannah, and a fierce lion approaches from a distance. You don't move, hoping it will leave you alone. It doesn't. It slowly walks right up to you, as tall as you are, and emanating low growls. As you stand there, afraid to run, it swipes a paw with claws extended. To your amazement, it has sliced through your clothes like butter, yet completely missed your flesh. Your clothes fall around you, and you haven't a scratch. The lion leans forward and you feel it's hot breath on your face as you fall backward into the soft grass. It steps forward until it is centered over you, and it slowly slides it's phallus into you. It begins to thrust faster and faster until it concludes with a roar that shakes the Earth.

Little Red Riding Hood

- *Husband = woodsman; Wife = Little Red Riding Hood;* You're running away from your Grandmother's house being chased by a wolf who intends to eat you. A woodsman comes to your rescue and kills the wolf. You let the woodsman eat you instead.

Lone Ranger

- *Husband = Lone Ranger; Wife = woman;* You're a pioneer woman out West and are accosted by outlaws who will surely use you to satisfy their lusts, when the Lone Ranger comes to your rescue. He takes you home, and you talk on the way. He takes you up on an offer to cook him a meal, and you become good friends. He comes by to check on you frequently, and your friendship blossoms into love. You find preacher and become the wife of the greatest hero in the West. Now you can finally give him every part of yourself, as you've wanted to do for so long.

Lord of the Manor

- *Husband = manor lord; Wife = servant;* You've been brought from the village to serve in the lord's manor, and it's been drilled into you that you must do whatever you're told. For weeks, you endure grueling tasks of scrubbing and cleaning. Then one evening you finally meet the lord, who is impressed with your beauty, and takes you to his chambers.

Lover & Beloved

From the Song of Solomon

- *Husband = lover; Wife = beloved;* You and your husband are the world's greatest lovers.

Mad Scientist

- *Husband = scientist; Wife = creature;* You come to life as a creature stitched together from many cadavers and sparked to life by a medical researcher. Your hormones must be out of balance, however, because all you can think about is sex.
- *Husband = scientist; Wife = creature;* You were killed in a car wreck, but an unconventional doctor took your

body home to his secret basement to experiment on your body. After several days he succeeds in bringing you back to life. He cannot let you leave his laboratory, however, because he would be imprisoned if his experiments were found out. Stuck there with no one else to talk to, you develop Stockholm Syndrome and make love to your hero/captor.

Option: Reverse roles.

Maid

- *Husband = employer; Wife = maid;* You're an upstairs maid and your uniform is an incredibly short French maid's outfit. You wouldn't mind it so much except that your employer finds it so erotic he drills you a few minutes every time he's around and you bend over for something. Although if you really minded, you might not be coming up with so many reasons to bend over...

Magician

- *Husband = subject; Wife = magician;* You create a love potion and pick a desirable single man to try it on. You get him to a restaurant, slip it into his drink, and it works extremely well. He can't think of anything but you, and he'll do anything you ask. Fortunately, once you get him home, his tongue and the rest of him are more than up to the job.
- *Husband = magician; Wife = subject;* You accept an invitation to a dinner party, but it turns out you're the only guest. You know you should leave, but find it very difficult. In fact, you find yourself staring into your host's eyes, and it becomes more and more difficult to control your thoughts or your body. After a few minutes, you are completely in his control. Anything he asks you to do, you want to do, and anything he tells you to do you are compelled to do. At first you experience some repulsion, but that fades as you become fixated on meeting your master's desires.

Masseuse

- *Husband = masseuse; Wife = client;* You 're enjoying your spa day and relax waiting for your full-body massage. The masseuse comes in, and you notice he locks the door behind him. Your concern vanishes as his hands soothe your muscles into a sublime rest. When you roll over and he works close to your breasts, you moan involuntarily. You open your eyes and notice that your nipples are very erect, then you notice your masseuse's eyes are as tender as his hands, and you moan intentionally to encourage his hands to explore every part of your breasts. As he gently kneads them, he slowly leans over and takes the closest nipple in his mouth. When he removes his mouth you feel disappointment, until you realize where he's moving it to.

- *Husband = client; Wife = masseuse;* You don't want to perform sex for money, but you want to do a good job as a masseuse, and that means the client should be very relaxed when you get through. You feel bad when your client gets a hard-on while you're massaging him, and you have a contradictory reluctance and compulsion to get him off. And this particular guy is so nice to you, and such a good tipper, and never complains...

Mentally Challenged

- *Husband = simple man; Wife = simple woman;* You and your best friend have no inhibitions, and enjoy each other's friendship more than anything else in life. And then you discover that touching each other can be a lot of fun.

Mermaid

- *Husband = man; Wife = mermaid;* You see the shadow of a ship on the surface and you swim up from the depths to see this rare sight. You are thrilled to see a man, and he seems to be as thrilled to see you. As the ship sails away, he watches you from the rear, then he jumps in and you swim toward each other. There, alone in the ocean, you swim together, stopping occasionally while he caresses your breasts as you kiss. You take him to the shore of a magical island, and you both sleep in the surf. When you awake you have legs like a woman, and the man delights in kissing you and licking you between them. The two of you slowly explore the island, eating its fruits and making endless love.

Mistress

- *Husband = man; Wife = mistress;* You were flattered at the attention of such a rich and powerful man, and surprised to learn that his wife was so uninterested in sex that she preferred he find someone else to satisfy his libido. During your intimate times together, you revel in such a great man's fondness for licking you into a frenzy, and you relish in the feelings of wealth and power you acquire by proxy when you satisfy him inside you.

Moses & Zipporah

Exodus 2:16-21

- *Husband = Moses; Wife = Zipporah;* You and your sisters are rescued by a strange man when trying to get water for your father's herd of sheep. Your father takes the stranger into his household, and you have fallen in love with him. You father has noticed your affection and arranged your marriage. Tonight, you share the stranger's bed for the first time.

Mountaineer

- *Husband = plane crash survivor; Wife = mountaineer widow:* You live alone in a cabin high in the mountains and are well prepared for the long winter that is just starting. A stranger staggers to your door just before a white-out hits. It's 20 miles to the nearest phone, and the snow will make it impossible to travel at all, possibly for weeks. His clothes are wet from having fallen into the creek outside your cabin, so you must get them off fast to keep him from hypothermia. He's too cold to help, and you need to rub your hands on any of his body parts you don't want to get frostbite. And... your cabin only has one bed.

Remember, you can always reverse roles.

Movie Star

- *Husband = movie star; Wife = fan;* You meet a famous movie star and he invites you to go with him to his hotel room. And he only has one thing on his mind.
- *Husband = fan; Wife = movie star;* You get interested in a guy at a party and take him to the closest bedroom.

- *Husband = producer; Wife = movie star;* You're up for a role in a new movie, and you meet with the producer in private to nail the part.

Mr. & Mrs. Kama Sutra

No, this wasn't really anyone's name.
- *Husband = Mr. Sutra; Wife = Mrs. Sutra;* You and your husband have written a bestselling book describing the most comprehensive set of sexual positions ever published. Now you have to find new ones for a sequel.

Mysterious Stranger

- *Husband = stranger; Wife = woman;* You meet a good looking man on a cross country train and discover he's witty and charming, but doesn't seem to be interested in coming to your compartment. He tells you he's getting off at the next stop to catch a plane to leave the country for good, but won't tell you why. You decide you really want him in your bed before he goes, so you ask him to come to your compartment to help you put a suitcase in an overhead bin. He obliges, and you seduce him as quickly as possible.

Newspaper Reporter

- *Husband = reporter; Wife = woman;* You're single and independent, and a good looking single reporter is referred to you as a possible subject for a human interest story. He finds you fascinating, and keeps taking you to dinner, supposedly to get more information for his story, but it obvious he has a very strong personal interest in you. You've never had anyone show so much appreciation in your personality, beliefs, and ideas, and you find him equally interesting. You invite him over to make dinner for him, supposedly to repay him for some of the dinners out, but once he starts kissing you, dinner will have to wait.

Nude Housekeeper

- *Husband = nude housekeeper; Wife = tenant:* You live alone in the big city and on a whim decide to try hiring a nude housekeeper to clean your apartment. It's a trial job, satisfaction guaranteed. It's silly, it's fun, and he does a good job of cleaning your bedroom and bathroom. And he's so good looking and good natured, you decide to ask him to clean your clock.

- *Husband = tenant; Wife = nude housekeeper:* You live alone in an efficiency apartment and on a whim decide to try hiring a nude housekeeper. She does a good job of cleaning and doesn't mind bending over to pick things up in a manner to give you an excellent view, from the front or rear. When she finishes the room, she eyes the bulge in your pants as she asks if there's anything else you want her to take care of.

Nun

- *Husband = young man; Wife = nun:* Your carriage breaks down on a stormy night and you approach the only chalet for miles around to seek refuge. You've never had difficulty with your vow of chastity until you met the lonely young man who has recently inherited his parents' estate. The two of you talk into the early morning, and find your interests are as one. After each he gets up to stoke the fire, get water, or some other task, he sits closer and closer, ending up by your side as he talks about his parents and begins to cry. You put an arm around him to comfort him, hoping that he doesn't respond physically, but he does. He pulls you close and embraces you, and your warming passion melts your reservations. As you savor your first kiss, you realize your several years of service is a life past, and as he caresses you, you look forward to a new life forever in his arms.

Nurse

- *Husband = patient; Wife = nurse:* You come on duty and find out that a good friend of yours was injured in a construction accident and is now a patient on your ward. He has a broken leg and some lacerations around his groin, and is being kept for observation. He came in dirty and can't get out of bed while the leg cast sets, so someone needs to give him a sponge bath and replace those bandages. There's only two other nurses on duty, and they're staying busy with other patients, so you reluctantly decide you must do the job.

Nymphomaniac

- *Husband = deliveryman; Wife = nympho:* Your sexual appetite is insatiable. You are compelled to have sex by any and every means possible with any male who crosses your path. Is that another deliveryman at the door?

You can try reversing the roles, but it's supposed to be exotic because it's rare, which doesn't work for a male in the nympho role since some people say this description applies to all men. ☺

Octoman

- *Husband = octoman: Wife = woman;* You've fallen in love with a man with a rare genetic defect: instead of arms and legs, he has 8 appendages with no bones that he can form into the shapes of arms, legs, cocks, and tongues. When you're in bed, you get lost in his caressing embrace and it's hard to tell where your body ends and his begins.

Oscar Winner

- *Husband = actor: Wife = date:* You're a last-minute date for an actor you've never heard of to take to the Oscars. Much to your surprise, he wins the Oscar for a category you weren't aware of: Best Actor in a Pornographic Leading Role. Hmm, maybe you can find out what makes him so good at that.

Outdoorsman

- *Husband = outdoorsman; wife = outdoorswoman;* You've gone for a hike in hilly forest and gotten lost, but are found by another hiker. Who offers to take you to his cabin since its almost dusk.

Painter (artistic)

- *Husband = painter: Wife = acquaintance:* You discover that your new friend is a very talented painter, and he invites you over to see his works. First you notice that all his works are nudes, then you notice that their style has a powerful way of conveying emotion. When he asks if you would pose for him, you blush and hesitate, but the request is too tempting to decline. He makes numerous sketches in an hour's time, and settles on one for an oil version. He shows them to you, and you're astonished that you look so beautiful in his eyes, and you agree to pose for the oil, though it will mean weeks of dedication. On your first sitting for the oil, he surprises you by telling you that you are the most beautiful woman he has ever known. He asks you to be his only model from now to the end of your lives, and he produces a ring which fits perfectly. You say yes, and you keep him far too busy to paint for days.

Paperboy

- *Husband = paperboy: Wife = customer's daughter:* You've developed a crush on the good-looking, hardworking boy who delivers your newspapers. You've figured out his monthly routine for coming by in the afternoons for payment, and you've been getting him to come into the house to wait while you look for the money despite knowing exactly where it was. Then you starting coming up with tasks for him to help you with, like moving something heavy, and he has always been very eager to help. He's due today, just after school, when you'll be alone in the house for at least an hour, and you plan to ask him up to your bedroom to help with something. Once in your room you'll reveal what you want help with: a kiss. You won't tell him that's just to get started... you'll let his body figure that out.

Pastor

- *Husband = pastor: Wife = woman;* You've gone through a bitter divorce despite years of pastoral counseling. Things were so bad you contemplated suicide more than once, but your widowed Pastor was a rock you could call on at any time. Late one night, you find yourself oppressed by your solitude and feel depression creeping back in. You call your Pastor in the middle of the night, and he takes you to an all night diner where you talk until morning. You've passed your crisis, and he takes you home again, and you fear he may be too sleepy to drive to his home, so you invite him in for coffee. You start the coffee as he gets cream out of the refrigerator, and you both turn and bump into each other. You look into each other's eyes, and the rest of the world disappears.

Pegasus & Ocyrhoe

- *Husband = Pegasus: Wife = Ocyrhoe;* You and your mate are winged horses, and only he is large enough to give you that wonderful feeling of fullness when he's inside you. You fly to the heights and soar in the warm thermal updrafts as your lover fills you with himself and you feel his hot seed enter you.

Personal Trainer

- *Husband = trainer: Wife = trainee:* You're trying to get in better shape, so you've hired a great-looking trainer to keep you going. After you finish your regular routine, he uses his tongue to get your heart rate up and breathing way up. Then you get in one last exercise and pay the bill at the same time by wildly swiveling your hips with his shaft inside you.
- *Husband = trainee: Wife = trainer:* You're paid to put this guy through a vigorous workout, starting with a tongue muscle endurance session with him laying face up on a bench and you straddling his face. Then it's time for him to practice his thrusting exercises.

Pilot

- *Husband = Pilot: Wife = target;* You meet an adrenaline-addicted Air Force jet-jockey who quickly becomes determined to conquer you. He drives a red convertible sports car and a big motorcycle, and you love riding with him. After several dates, your resistance is beginning to wear thin and you start thinking about the possible need for birth control when he really catches you off guard: a dinner invitation turns out to include a surprise cross-country flight to Seattle in a friend's private jet. There in the restaurant at the top of the Space Needle, he admits that he initially only wanted to have sex with you and move on, but that he has fallen completely in love with you. He gets down on his knee and proposes as a bevy of waiters appear and surround your table, each bearing a dozen red roses. You accept, and soon take your new groom-to-be to the closest hotel. It's your fertile period so there's a danger of getting pregnant before you actually get married, but you can also enjoy an occasional adrenaline rush. Then

he asks you if you want to fly to Las Vegas in the
morning and get married right away.

Pirate

- *Husband = Pirate: Wife = Governor's daughter;* You're
  taken captive by a remarkably interesting pirate so he
  can demand a ransom for your return. You have a
  demand of your own.

Plumber

- *Husband = home-owner: Wife = plumber;* You're
  called again to the home of your favorite customer, a
  great-looking single guy with a great personality and
  sense of humor, and prosperous enough to own his own
  home. You've started wondering about his back luck,
  though, as his house has had one problem after another.
  This time it is clear that someone has intentionally
  sabotaged the pipes. Hmm. And he lives alone, so that
  means... you turn around to go confront him, and he's
  standing there watching with a grin on his mug. He
  apologizes half-heartedly for the deceit and you just
  stand there not knowing what to say. You're in messy
  work duds, and he steps closer and says you're
  beautiful. You stammer that you haven't washed your
  hair in several days and a couple of sprigs of hair dangle
  in your face. The two of you talk as you fix what he
  broke. Then he ends up washing your hair, and you
  decide you're going to take care of all his plumbing
  needs from then on.

Pocahontas & John Rolfe

- *Husband = John Rolfe: Wife = Princess Pocahontas;*
  You are the princess of a powerful Indian chief, and you
  fall in love with a European settler in Jamestown. You
  get married despite either of you being fluent in the
  other's language, and now it's your wedding night. And
  you have no trouble communicating your desires.

Politician

- *Husband = politician: Wife = voter;* It's election time
  again, and you've met a pol who will literally do
  anything you ask in order to get your vote.

Sexual Fantasy Cookbook: Sex Recipes
See "Fantasy vs. Lust" beginning on page 95.

President & Bimbo

- *Husband = President: Wife = bimbo;* You visit the President in the oval office, and he takes you into an adjoining hallway where there are no cameras. He gets to relieve his sex drive, and you get to have the most powerful man in the world inside you.

Priest

- *Husband = Priest: Wife = penitent;* You're a young, naïve woman who goes to a Catholic Church to confess your sins. Unfortunately, the Priest tending the confessional is obsessed with sex and tells you that you have to do penance by going into a back room with him and doing whatever he tells you.

Prostitute, Coarse

- *Husband = customer: Wife = prostitute;* You're all business. You collect the money up front, strip, suck, and fuck. Next...
- *Husband = prostitute: Wife = customer;* Your "escort" is all business. He demands his money up front, strips you and licks you off. Next...

Prostitute, New

- *Husband = customer: Wife = prostitute;* You've never done this before and you're timid and reserved.

Don't forget you can reverse any roles!

Prostitute, Desperate

- *Husband = customer: Wife = prostitute;* You're so desperate you'll do anything for some money. Even after making the big decision to have sex for money, it seems to take forever to try to find a customer. You're determined to do whatever he asks and pretend you enjoy it so maybe he'll give you a big tip.

Prostitute, Refined

- *Husband = customer: Wife = prostitute;* You're elegant and sophisticated, and *very* expensive. One advantage of having a high price is that you have very few customers, and they're generally very rich, powerful men. Today you're breaking in a new client.

Prostitute, Elite

- *Husband = customer: Wife = prostitute;* You're the expert all the other girls come to for advice on how to satisfy men with a variety of desires and expectations. And your clients are all repeat customers who can't get enough of you – because you're that good.

Queen

- *Husband = chamberlain: Wife = Queen;* You work hard all day ruling the entire country, while your titular husband spends most of his time behind closed doors with a variety of courtiers. A minor Prince in his homeland, you've never been intimate with your husband, whom you took to ensure peace between your country and his native country, and he has never shown any interest in you. Fortunately for you, the chamberlain you chose to manage your household is as capable in meeting your physical needs as he is in taking care of the other servants.

Rahab

Joshua 2:1-7, 6:17-25
- *Husband = spy: Wife = Rahab;* You're a professional prostitute and very bright. You've heard of the exploits of the people invading your land, and you foresee that it's inevitable that they will conquer your city. Your cheap apartment is built into the outer wall, quite vulnerable if that portion of the wall is attacked. You plan to take refuge elsewhere in the city when the time comes, but then are surprised when one of the invaders' spies comes to your door to escape the city guards. You offer to protect him in exchange for a promise of safety when the city falls, and he agrees. You look out the door and see the guards coming, so you decide to hide the spy in plain sight – by quickly stripping his clothes and getting busy in bed. The ploy works, as the guards look in and quickly excuse themselves. Well... you might as well finish what you started.

Repairman

- *Husband = repairman: Wife = businesswoman:* You've had to take a half day of vacation because your condo's roof has started leaking, and the repairman needs to get into your attic to determine where the leak is coming from. You're surprised when his van pulls up on time, and you think maybe you can just work a little late tonight and save your vacation time. Then he gets out, and your body starts talking louder than your brain. Maybe you should take a whole day of vacation. He gets into the attic and calls out to you, but you can't understand what he's saying. Then he crashes through the ceiling right onto your bed. "I said I found the leak", he says, unhurt, but having this man on your bed is more than you can stand. You might need two days of vacation.

Robot

- *Husband = robot: Wife = owner;* You are the proud new owner of a robot servant with artificial intelligence, voice control, and full sexual capabilities. Try him out – he can't say no.
- *Husband = owner: Wife = robot;* You are a robot with artificial intelligence and you become self-aware when your new owner gets you home and activates you for the first time. You are a model full capable of fulfilling all sexual requests and you are programmed to fulfill your owners voice commands without hesitation. You only ask questions in order to clarify requests.

Rock star

- *Husband = rock star; Wife = groupie:* You can't believe your luck to get picked out of the crowd to go back stage to the star's dressing room after the concert. He makes it clear from the start that he's only interested in one thing. That's exactly what you expected and wanted, and you plan to do that thing better than anyone he's ever done it with before.
- *Husband = stage hand; Wife = rock star:* You finished a big set and had the crowd chanting your name – what a rush! Now you're back in your hotel room and its emptiness seems oppressive and inappropriate for someone as famous as you. A stage hand found your wallet back stage while putting the equipment away and has come to your door to return it. You give him reward that he could only have dreamed of.

Ruth & Boaz

Ruth 2-4

- *Husband = Boaz: Wife = Ruth;* You fall in love with your protector and relative (distant enough to be a legal husband), and you ask him to marry you by going into his bedroom and getting under the covers. He loves you, and as difficult as it is, he keeps his hands off until he clears the marriage with another male relative who has a claim on you. They work it out and now it's your wedding night. This time when you share his bed, there will be lots and lots of touching.

Samson & Delilah

Judges 14-16

- *Husband = Samson: Wife = Delilah;* You have to seduce a warrior and get him to confide a secret to try to protect your family from the ruthless ruler of your people. Fortunately, your victim is enamored with you.

Santa Claus

- *Husband = Santa Claus; wife = bad girl;* Ho, ho, ho! Santa Clause has just come down the chimney in the middle of the night, and you're not letting him leave until you give him your present!

Secretary

- *Husband = businessman; wife = secretary;* You admire your powerful, influential, good-looking single boss, but he seems to think of you only for your office skills. You want to get him to think of much more than that.
- *Husband = businessman; wife = secretary;* Your powerful, influential boss can do a lot for your career, and you want to get him in bed and get pictures for leverage.
- *Husband = businessman; wife = secretary;* You and your boss travel to another city together, but the hotel messed up the reservation and only has one room with one bed.
- *Husband = businessman; wife = secretary;* You and your boss travel to another city together and your hotel rooms have an adjoining door that won't lock. You can't resist sneaking into his room in the middle of the night.

Option: Reverse the roles to make the wife run the business and have the husband be the secretary.

Sex Therapist

- *Husband = man; wife = sex therapist;* Your practice is talk-only therapy, and you've been working with a male patient who had been able to masturbate before marriage, but had never been able to attain an erection while married. Extensive testing showed no physical problems. His wife refused to attend any sessions, left him, and filed for a divorce which was recently finalized. The patient has requested the continuation of therapy in order to try to overcome his problem so that he might pursue marriage again after he has improved. After the divorce, he reluctantly began to reveal negative traits about his ex-wife, specifically that she was an extremely controlling, demanding, and obsessive person. For a second time, you suggest he try walking in the woods as a relaxation technique, and this time he promises to try that. But then he leaves a voice mail abruptly canceling all his scheduled sessions and says that he no longer wishes to be your patient. He provides no explanation, which leaves you feeling a little unfulfilled. So the following Saturday, you go for a walk in the woods, which is one of your own favorite ways to relax. And there in the middle of the forest, you run into your former patient. You express surprise, and he reminds you that you told him about how you enjoy walking in these very woods. And he didn't just come to relax... he came to wait for you. Your mind quickly runs through many issues: he is officially no longer a patient, he's single, he's about your age, he's great looking, he's got a great personality, he... he steps up to you and kisses you. Oh! He's... a very good kisser. He puts his arms around you and pulls you to him, and he... no longer has a problem getting an erection! Fight or flight: your brain demands a decision! It's been a long time since your husband died, and to your surprise, you feel completely comfortable in his arms. Your decision is to... relax, and melt into his embrace. The two of you spend hours walking and talking, and then kissing again. Lost in happiness, you take him by the hand well off the trail, and completely hidden by the many trees, consummate your new non-professional relationship.

Sex Toy Demonstrator

- *Husband = demonstrator; wife = customer;* You go into a sex toy store for the first time and are mystified at all the products. A handsome salesman offers to demonstrate them to you or on you right there in the store.
- *Husband = demonstrator; wife = customer;* You go into a sex toy store for the first time and are mystified at all the products. You ask the handsome salesman to bring some to your house to demonstrate them in person.

Shape-Shifter

- *Husband = shape-shifter: Wife = woman;* You're a botanist exploring the flora on a new planet and get far from your team. There's no chance of getting lost with all your gadgets, and you enjoy the solitude and the environment, which is so much like Earth. Until an unfamiliar human male appears in a team uniform, but he is definitely not part of your team. He speaks your language perfectly and welcomes you to his home. Then you realize he looks like a science teacher you had a crush on in high school, and he explains that he took his current form based on ideas from your mind! He illustrates by shifting his appearance to another man from your past, then several more. In a flash, your mind remembers having sex with your beloved but deceased husband, and wonder if... The creature's shape changes again and now looks like your husband, with no clothes, and a prominent erection. Your gasp involuntarily. You want to turn your gaze away, but cannot. You stare as he sits on a moss-like step and tells you about his planet, his people, his culture, and himself/itself. In the form of your husband, you feel at ease, and rejoin the conversation by telling him all about Earth, your exploration effort, yourself, and your husband. You digress into the sex life you had before he died, and the creature is fascinated. He asks what if feels like, and as you try to describe it, he reaches out and tenderly strokes your arm, sending shivers down your back. Reading thoughts in your mind you'd rather he not, he continues to touch you in more and more intimate places.

Sexual Fantasy Cookbook: Sex Recipes
See "Fantasy vs. Lust" beginning on page 95.

Slave Master

- *Husband = slave; wife = slave master;* You manage all the slaves working to pay off debts and are responsible for assigning them their tasks. All want to stay in your good graces, but some are willing to go further than others.

Remember, you can always reverse the roles.

Sleeping Beauty

- *Husband = the prince; wife = Sleeping Beauty;* Put into a 100 year sleep when your finger is pricked by an enchanted spindle, the only way to revive you is for a prince to prick you with his enchanted cock, causing you both to fall in love with each other forever. You awaken with him inside you and know that he loves you with all his heart, and you wish the that moment would last 100 years.

Snow White

- *Husband = the prince and all 7 dwarfs; wife = Snow White;* In this world, women can have as many husbands as they desire. You hold the record, and regularly enjoy satisfying one after another, after another, after another...

Soldier

- *Husband = soldier; wife = fiancée;* Your fiancée was called to duty in a military unit that will be heading to the front lines immediately, and it unlikely he will survive. You get married immediately and have one chance to get pregnant before he has to leave.
- *Husband = soldier; wife = citizen;* You're a citizen that is occupied by a foreign army, and a soldier fighting for your country's freedom has been stranded behind the lines. You find him hiding outside your house in the cold, and you bring him in to feed him , get him warm, and give him a better hiding place. You get scared when the artillery gets closer and the power is knocked out, and your hero comforts you, and all inhibitions fade away.
- *Husband = soldier; wife = victim;* Your village is overrun by an invading army and as a beautiful single

girl, you are one of the prize spoils of war. The leader gives you to one of his best warriors.

Spiderman

- *Husband = Spiderman: Wife = Mary Jane;* You had a boyfriend. It developed into love. You got married. It's your wedding night. He left 3 hours ago with no explanation, and he's just come back. His defense? He's Spiderman, and his spidy-sense detected trouble requiring his intervention. He proves it to you and apologizes that he hid the truth from you until now. He offers to take you back to your parents and get an annulment if you want it. Now you know everything, and you have to decide what happens next.

Spy

- *Husband = spy; wife = diplomat;* You have information highly desire by a foreign government, and a debonair spy is trying to seduce you to get it. He won't get the info, but you'll have fun getting what you want from him.
- *Husband = government worker; wife = spy;* It has been determined that a particular man knows certain classified information and you've been assigned to seduce him and get him to confide the information to you. Your plan is to give him great sex, and make him think that's he's giving you great sex, so great that he'll do absolutely anything to keep you happy.
- *Husband = spy; wife = foreigner;* A strange man lunges as you get into your car and forces you into the passenger seat at gun-point as he gets in and drives wildly away. A gun-shot through your back window is more than sufficient evidence that someone is after the guy. As he races through the streets, he apologizes and explains that he's from your native country and he has information critical to its national security. Unfortunately, because those chasing him may have seen your car's tag number, your life is now in danger. He loses the tail, finds a cheap motel and hides the car to wait until he can reach his escape contact tomorrow, promising to take you to safety with him. After noting that the room only has one bed, you decide to give your sexy spy some extra incentive to keep you safe.

Stable hand

- *Husband = stable hand; wife = equestrian;* You've just returned to the stable after a wonderfully long horseback ride in the countryside. As you dismount, the stable hand arrives to take your horse, and his nearness causes you to realize how aroused you became from the rhythmic pounding you experienced during your ride. You follow the stable hand and help him put the horse away, then you mount up again.

Statue

- *Husband = statue: Wife = woman;* You get horny and decide to relieve yourself so you climb down the stairs into the basement where there is a full-sized statue of a nude man with a fully erect penis, laying on its back. It was chiseled out of the bedrock by the old woman who owned the house before you. You got the house cheap because the old woman died in the house, but you didn't care about that because you could not stop imagining how you would make use of your statue, which you named "Major Pike". Once again, you remove the dust sheet to expose the Major and lower yourself onto its hard, unyielding treasure.

Stowaway

- *Husband = chief steward: Wife = stowaway;* You fled a life of misery in a war-torn, heartless country and snuck aboard a ship bound for America, but lost your bag of toiletries in doing so. You have to come out of hiding periodically to steal food and drink, and use a toilet. You go into a stateroom's private bath looking for some pads or a substitute, but get caught by the ship's chief steward. He only speaks English, which you don't speak at all. He apparently intends to arrest you, but with great embarrassment you try to use gestures to explain your needs. You notice he has no wedding ring, and wonder if he knows about menstruation, but he finally seems to figure out what you mean. He leaves you in his room and comes back with pads, and lets you use his bathroom. When you finally come out, he surprises you by letting you stay in his room. He removes some personal items and he returns often to bring you hot food. You begin sharing meals, and your appreciation for his kindness grows into trust, and then love. After one evening meal, you try to get him to stay with you.

Superman

- *Husband = Superman: Wife = Lois;* You finally learn Superman's true identity when he proposes, and you accept. When you get in bed with him the first time, you warn him not to get so carried away that he forgets how strong he is. But say, just how fast is his tongue?

Survivors

- *Husband = survivor; Wife = survivor:* You were relaxing in a nice hot bath in a luxury hotel when an earthquake hit. You figure the tub is as safe as anywhere else, so you plan to ride out the shaking in the tub, but then the hotel collapses and the lights go out. It's pitch black, and you feel around and discover sheet rock on top of the tub and concrete not much above that. You crawl out though an opening barely big enough to squeeze through. You explore as far as you can reach, but you feel no towels, clothes, or anything clothe-like, although you feel several spaces that are big enough to try crawling through. You hear moaning right below you. A man had been taking a shower and was knocked unconscious, but seems okay now. You start talking and discover he was in the room right below yours. He feels around and only has one avenue of escape, which brings him into your space. The two of you spend hours crawling around in the dark, and determine that you're trapped in a space that has the remnants of your bathroom, a tiny space where his bathtub was, and a space with part of a mattress that's not covered by concrete. Heated until now by the exertions of your searching, you both start to get tired and cold. The only logical thing to do is to share the partial mattress and body heat. And his body heat feels sooo good, you want more and more.

Teacher

- *Husband = high school teacher; Wife = student;* You're a high school student with a huge crush on your teacher and you won't rest until you experience his body. You study his habits and catch him alone one day after

Sexual Fantasy Cookbook: Sex Recipes
See "Fantasy vs. Lust" beginning on page 95.

school in the teacher's lounge. He tries to get away from you until you get him cornered and get your hand in his pants. He's temporarily too shocked to react, you follow up by immediately getting his pants loose and putting your mouth on him. That shuts down his higher brain functions and until you're done, he's little more than a real-life sex toy.

- *Husband = college professor; Wife = student;* Forget sex for grades, you want the stud teaching your class in your bed even though you can get an A on your own.
- *Husband = student; Wife = high school teacher;* It's your first year teaching and the age difference between you and the seniors isn't that great. And there's one boy who seems as interested in you as you are in him. He readily accepts when you ask him to come over to your apartment to move some heavy boxes... off the bed.
- *Husband = student; Wife = college professor;* You pride yourself on your extensive knowledge in your field, but this one older-than-usual study has an annoying habit of asking questions that stump you. Until he takes you to lunch at the cafeteria and reveals that's he's studied you intensely to determine just where your weaknesses might be. Justly flattered, your friendship depends after the semester ends and he ends up at your house late one evening, having had too much wine to drive home safely. But not too much to be very romantic.
- *Husband = high school teacher; Wife = high school teacher:* There's a bed left behind the stage from the school's last play, and it's very isolated. Perfect for a rendezvous on your prep period.

Tenant
- *Husband = tenant; Wife = tenant;* You live in an apartment building in New York City, and you're anxious to meet your new, good-looking single neighbor across the hall. You finally meet in the elevator, just as the power goes out for hours.

Time Traveler
- *Husband = politician; Wife = time traveler;* You travel back in time to learn about your great-grandfather, a doctor, and your great-grandmother. Much is known in

the future about him, but few records have ever been found of his wife, who you were named after. You arrive a few days before they first met, find your great-grandfather, and begin stealthily following him each day. Once he meets her, you plan to start following her until you can document her past. The next day you're following him on a crowed sidewalk, lose sight of him and start to panic. You run ahead, looking in all directions, and are startled when you run right into him. He turns as you fall and your head hits the concrete hard. When you wake, you're in a hospital with a terrible headache and you can only remember your name. An exceptionally nice doctor tells you he brought you to his hospital after you fell and hit your head. He dotes on you as you recover and you both fall madly in love.

Touchstone

Passive version

- *Husband = man; Wife = Touchstone;* You're "The Touchstone", and no one in your world is capable of sexual pleasure until their libido is activated by having sex with you, which has the effect of turning on their sexual hormone glands.

Active version

- *Husband = Touchstone; Wife = woman;* You are incapable of sexual pleasure or becoming pregnant until The Touchstone brings you to your first orgasm, which will initiate the glands that produce your sexual hormones.

Option: Reverse roles.

Transformed Animal

- *Husband = dog; Wife = owner:* Your husband took your dog for a walk and lightening struck them, transferring their consciousnesses. Your husband, going into the dog and thereby being limited to a dog brain, ran off with other dogs. Your dog, going into your husband's body, doesn't know how to use the extra parts of its new brain, so it acts just like the old dog. You and your dog (in your husband's old body) miss your husband, and you let the dog sleep curled up on the end of the bed. Well, maybe something of your husband is left, because the dog sure likes licking you.

Choose any type of animal

- *Husband = man; Wife = animal;* You're in heat and can't think about anything except getting a male to impregnate you. While in the condition, you transform into the species of whatever kind of male is closest. You cannot speak the language of other species, but that's never stopped a male from humping you. You sniff the scent of a male of some kind and follow it straight into a house. Now you sense a male very close and begin to transform, and your pheromones are starting to put the male into sexual frenzy.

Option: Reverse roles.

Traveling Salesman

- *Husband = traveling salesman; Wife = housewife;* You answer the door to find a handsome door-to-door salesman selling sex toys. You invite him in to show you how they all work.
- *Husband = traveling salesman; Wife = farmer's daughter;* You've been stuck on the farm ever since you hit puberty, and you can't wait to get alone with a man and find out what sex is like. When a traveling salesman comes to your house, you slip him a note asking him to drive away and come back to meet you in the barn. He shows up right on time, and you start making up for lost time.

Truck Driver

- *Husband = truck driver; Wife = hitchhiker;* You're traveling cross country and accept a ride from a nice trucker. You enjoy each other's company so much you decide to just wherever he's going. In fact, you like him so much, you decide to go wherever he's going from now on, including when he crawls into the back bunk.
- *Husband = truck driver; Wife = waitress;* There aren't many good paying jobs in your neck of the woods, but as a waitress at a trucks stop, you can supplement your income in the back of truckers' cabs. And you need some extra cash now...

Sexual Fantasy Cookbook: Sex Recipes
See "Fantasy vs. Lust" beginning on page 95.

Umpire
- *Husband = umpire; Wife = athlete:* Your team is behind and won't win without help, so you call a time-out, walk over to the umpire, pull his pants down, drop your pants and bend over. After that, the calls all go your team's way.
- *Husband = athlete; Wife = umpire:* You call a foul, and the person you call it on walks over, gets down on his knees, puts his head under your skirt, pulls your panties aside and gives you a tongue-lashing. You decide to reverse your call.

Valet
No, not parking valet, just valet, which means "personal man-servant".
- *Husband = valet; Wife = lady of the house:* You climb to the top of the highest tower of your mansion and summon your valet and make him service you from behind as you survey your land from horizon to horizon.

Vampire
- *Husband = vampire; Wife = woman;* You wake up in bed with a strange man in the room. You want to scream, but his mind is exerting too much control over you. You skin feels like he is touching you all over, even though you see him standing with his arms to his side. He tells you that he is a vampire, but not like in the movies. He requires the special juices from a human female's pussy, and when he drinks it, it gives him power and makes the woman his slave forever. He removes the sheets and your sleeping clothes and you cannot move... until his tongue starts licking your clitoris to force your vagina to produce lubrication, and you start moving and moaning. You cannot refrain from an orgasm, which is out-of-this-world/out-of-your-mind incredible. Perhaps being his eternal love-slave won't be so bad.

Widow / Widower
- *Husband = widower; Wife = widow:* Your body may be old, but your libido is as healthy as ever. When an eligible widower moves next door, you decide to find out how strong his libido is.

- 266 -

Sexual Fantasy Cookbook: Sex Recipes
See "Fantasy vs. Lust" beginning on page 95.

Werewolf

- *Husband = werewolf; Wife = woman:* You fell in love with a man with a dark, mysterious side, but you actually found that attractive. The night before your wedding he came to you and told you his darkest secret to give you a chance to change your mind about the marriage. His secret: he is a werewolf, and he has to chain himself up at every full moon, or the rage he experiences while transformed would surely cause him to kill anyone and anything he could. And you thought your period was bad. You marry him anyway, primarily because you love him, and partly because you doubt it could be true. The truth of the matter became plain on your wedding night, however, as your virgin groom and you discovered together that he partially transforms during sex, although when he transforms because of sexual excitement, he doesn't suffer from rage, and he transforms back immediately afterward. And it's quite a wild experience for you.

X-Husband & X-Wife

- *Husband = ex-husband; Wife = ex-wife:* You were frustrated by your marriage and happy when it ended, but you've missed the sex terribly. When you meet each other again at a dinner party, you dance together and your passions become irresistible and very impatient. The two of you sneak upstairs to one of the hosts' bedrooms to and have passionate sex.
- *Husband = ex-husband; Wife = ex-wife:* You always regretted that things didn't work out with your husband, and were inwardly pleased to hear that he was still single. When you meet again, you both discover you still have desire for each other and you have more respect for each other than you had before. You decide to go on a date, then another, then another. Tonight the only argument is where the two of you will spend the night together.

Yankee in King Arthur's Court

- *Husband = Yankee; Wife = courtier:* You are amazed at the brashness of this strange Yankee who speaks his mind frankly without deference to nobility. You decide to see if he's equally brash in bed.

- *Husband = king; Wife = Yankee:* You travel through time and space to the time before King Arthur meets Guinevere, and he is enchanted by your candor and spunk. You are unlike any woman he has ever known, and he is captivated as you lead him into his tent alone.

Zipper

- *Husband = Zipper: Wife = woman;* You're single and occasionally hire Zipper, the fastest tongue in the West. Not much for talking, he just gets the job done and disappears.

Zorro

- *Husband = Zorro; Wife = woman in danger:* You are walking home through the streets late at night in a Mexican city long ago, having helped your cousin give birth. Too exhausted to be vigilant, you are accosted by rogue soldiers who mean to have their way with you before they leave your lifeless body in the gutter. You scream and fight back, but they're too strong. Your clothes are ripped from you and one man holds each arm and leg, legs spread apart, waiting to treat another soldier lucky enough to have you first. Except a sword tip appears through his chest. As he falls, Zorro is revealed behind him. The other soldiers drop you and draw their swords. At four against one, it's not a fair fight. Faster than the blink of an eye, one is pierced through the heart, then the next soldier's thrust is parried and his artery is severed. The third and fourth men duel Zorro for a fleeting moment before their lives come to an end. Zorro bends kneels by you and raises you to a sitting position while his sword tip picks what remains of your clothes off the ground. He delivers them to your hands, and you cover yourself as best you can with them. When he gets you home, you learn his secret: He is none other than the man you are engaged to marry. You decide not to wait to demonstrate your profound love.

Remember to stir your creativity. You can reverse roles by gender-reversal role-playing or by redefining the roles. For example, you can rewrite Zorro to become Zorrette!

Sexual Fantasy Cookbook: Sex Recipes

See "Fantasy vs. Lust" beginning on page 95.

Pick a letter, any letter...

We've got at least one fantasy scenario for every letter in the English alphabet. Pick a letter at random to help you choose which fantasy to try next!

[Use this blank space for notes about your own fantasy ideas!]

[Use this blank space for notes about your own fantasy ideas!]

RECOMMENDED READING

Other books & reading material recommended by Grandma:

The Act of Marriage, The Beauty of Sexual Love
Tim & Beverly LaHaye, Zondervan, Michigan, 1976

Ask Alice (Columbia University)
http://www.goaskalice.columbia.edu/Cat6.html

Best Friends For Life
Michael & Judy Phillips, Bethany House, Minnesota, 1997

The Complete Idiot's Guide to The Kama Sutra
Johanina Wikoff, Ph.D. and Deborah S. Romaine
Alpha Books, Indianapolis, 2000

The Five Love Languages: How to Express Heartfelt Commitment to Your Mate
Gary Chapman, Northfield Publishing, Chicago, 1995

Gift Wrapped by God
By Linda Dillow & Lorraine Pintus, WaterBrook Press, Colorado, 2004

He Comes Next: The Thinking Woman's Guide to Pleasuring a Man
Ian Kerner, Ph.D., Collins Living, 2006

How To Make Love To A Man
By Alexandra Penney, Wing Books, New York, 1980

How To Make Love To A Woman
By Michael Morgenstern, Diadem Books, New York, 1982

Intended for Pleasure: Sex Technique and Sexual Fulfillment in Christian Marriage
Ed Wheat and Gaye Wheat, Revell, Michigan, 1997

Intimacy Ignited
By Dr. Jody & Linda Dillow and Dr. Peter & Lorraine Pintus, NavPress, Colorado, 2004

Intimate Issues
By Linda Dillow & Lorraine Pintus, WaterBrook Press, Colorado, 1999

Lord of Life, Lord of Me
Bill Ameiss and Jane Craver, Condordia, St. Louis, 1982

Ride 'Em Cowgirl! Sex Position Secrets For Better Bucking
Dr. Sadie Allison, Tickle Kitty Press, 2007

Sex God: Exploring the Endless Connections between Sexuality and Spirituality
Rob Bell, Zondervan, Michigan, 2008

She Comes First: The Thinking Man's Guide to Pleasuring a Woman
Ian Kerner, Ph.D., Collins Living, 2004

Solomon On Sex, The Biblical Guide to Married Love
Joseph C. Dillow, Thomas Nelson Publishers, New York, 1977

A Song For Lovers
S. Craig Glickman, Intervarsity Press, Illinois, 1976

Tickle His Pickle: Your Hands-On Guide to Penis Pleasing
Dr. Sadie Allison, Tickle Kitty Press, 2004

The World's Easiest Guide to Family Relationships
Gary Chapman, Northfield Publishing, Chicago, 2001

GLOSSARY OF SEXUAL TERMS

Adultery, when one or both of the people having sex are married to someone other than the person they are having sex with.

A-Spot (Anterior Fornix), a female erogenous zone, the deepest point on the front wall of the vagina located between the cervix and the bladder.

Anal Beads, a sex toy for insertion into the anus.

Anus, external opening of the rectum. It has many nerve endings, making it an erogenous zone for both men and women.

Arousal, the process of getting ready for sexual activity and feeling an urge for sexual contact.

Ass, slang for anus.

Balls, slang for testicles.

Balls-to-Chin, another term for deep-throating.

Balls-to-the-Walls, slang for "maximum thrust" (from the aviation term), or a penis that is fully inserted into a woman's vagina, anus, or mouth.

Bang, slang for vaginal or anal intercourse.

Beaver, slang for vagina.

Blow Job, slang for fellatio.

Bondage, the use of physical restraints in sexual fantasies.

Bonding, creating or strengthening an emotional attachment to another person.

Boner, slang for erect penis.

Bonk, slang for vaginal or anal intercourse.

Boobs, slang for breasts.

Buff, slang for naked or muscular.

Bush, pubic hair or slang for vagina.

Butt Plug, a sex toy for insertion into the anus.

Cameltoe, slang for a woman's public mound when covered by very tight cloth, such as a swimsuit.

Carpet, slang for a woman whose participation in sex is totally passive.

Chaste, a synonym for virgin.

Cherry, slang for the vagina of a virgin.

Clit, short for clitoris.

Clitoris, a female sexual organ, the only known purpose of which is to induce sexual pleasure.

Climax, another word for orgasm.

Cock, slang for penis.

Cock Ring, a sex toy that encircles the penis and is used to delay ejaculation and heighten pleasure.

Cream, slang for semen.

Condom, a covering for the penis that is used to reduce the likelihood of pregnancy or transfer of a sexual disease.

Contraception, any of numerous methods of trying to prevent pregnancy despite having sexual intercourse.

Costume Token, a small piece of a full costume, used to enhance the imagination during role-playing.

Cum, slang for orgasm or semen.

Cumming, slang for orgasm or imminent orgasm.

Cunnilingus, oral sex performed on a woman.

Cunt, slang for vagina. Also used in a very derogatory manner to refer to a woman, implying that she has no value other than her vagina.

Dead Fish, slang for a woman whose participation in sex is totally passive.

Deep Throat, slang for fellatio in which the penis is inserted in the mouth beyond the epiglottis and into the throat.

Dick, slang for penis.

Dong, slang for penis.

Double Penetration (DP), simultaneous penetration of a woman's vagina and her anus.

Drill, slang for vaginal or anal intercourse.

Eating Pussy, slang for cunnilingus.

Ejaculation, the ejection of semen from the penis, usually accompanied by orgasm.

Erotic, anything that arouses or satisfies sexual desire.

Erotic Literature, narrative text intended to arouse sexual feelings, analogous to a visual version usually referred to as pornography.

Erotica, sexually arousing nudity without explicit sexual intercourse, in any form of media (writing, video, picture, video game, sculpture, etc).

Erogenous Zone, an area of the human body with heightened sensitivity, the stimulation of which normally results in a sexual response.

Facial, slang for a man ejaculating on a woman's face.

Fingering, slang for stimulating the clitoris with a finger or fingers.

Fisting, inserting an entire hand into a vagina or anus.

Fellatio, oral sex performed on a man.

Fetish, an erotic fixation on an object or non-genital body part.

Foreplay, sexually oriented activity ranging from very mildly erotic (e.g., talking, teasing, hugging) to anything just short of sexual intercourse or oral sex.

Fornication, sex between 2 unmarried people.

French Kiss, a form of kissing in which at least one spouse inserts their tongue in the other's mouth, simulating intercourse.

Friends With Benefits, slang for a friend you have casual sex with on a regular basis.

Fuck/Fucking, slang for vaginal intercourse.

Fuck-Buddy, slang for a friend you have casual sex with on a regular basis.

Fucking Machine, a motorized sex toy that thrusts a dildo or butt plug in and out.

G-Spot (Gräfenberg Spot), a patch of rough tissue along the front of the vaginal canal, with a texture similar to the palate (the roof of a mouth). It is not be present in all women, and though it is known as a female erogenous zone, it's erogenous effect may come from stimulation of the paraurethral gland near it.

GLOSSARY

Gangbang, slang for an orgy with multiple simultaneous sex partners.

Getting Laid, slang for having intercourse.

Getting Off, slang for having an orgasm.

Giving Head, slang for oral sex.

Going Down, slang for oral sex.

Gonads, another word for testicles.

Hand Job, slang for using the hands to stimulate a penis or clitoris.

Hardcore, pornography that shows explicit sexual intercourse.

Hard-on, slang for erection.

Harness, straps used to hold a dildo or clitoral vibrator in position.

Horny, slang for being sexually aroused of having an erection.

Hosing, slang for a woman masturbating by aiming a water stream on the clitoris.

Hooters, slang for breasts.

Hump/Humping, slang for vaginal or anal intercourse.

Hump-Rub, a technique that combines the husband thrusting in and out while the wife uses a finger or vibrator on her clitoris. This is the best way to try to achieve simultaneous orgasm for many couples.

Inner Thigh, an erogenous zone, primarily for women.

Jack-Off, slang for masturbation, especially by males.

Jerk-Off, slang for masturbation, especially by males.

Jewels, slang for testicles.

Jism, slang for semen.

Jizz, slang for semen.

Jugs, slang for breasts.

Kegel Exercise, a method of improving pubococcygeus muscle tone in the pelvic floor, which can increase sexual pleasure.

Kiss, one person touching another person with their lips. Between spouses, this is often lips-to-lips.

Knockers, slang for breasts.

Lascivious, dominated by uninhibited sexual desires.

Licking out, slang for cunnilingus.

Love Language, one of 5 ways identified by Dr. Gary Chapman that people show and perceive love: encouraging words, physical touch, physical gifts, quality time, or acts of service. (See http://www.fivelovelanguages.com/learn.html)

Lubricant, a fluid inserted into the vagina or anus, or applied to the penis, to reduce friction and dryness.

Mammary Intercourse, enclosing or partial enclosing the husband's penis between the wife's breasts.

Masturbation, manually stimulating one's own genitals, usually to the point of orgasm. Sometimes used to refer to any use of hands to stimulate a spouse's genitals.

Melons, slang for breasts.

Moustache Ride, slang for cunnilingus.

MILF, "Mother I'd Like to Fuck", slang for a sexually attractive older woman.

Muff, slang for vagina.

Muff Diving, slang for cunnilingus.

Nail, slang for vaginal or anal intercourse.

Multi-Orgasmic, an immediate return to the plateau phase after an orgasm so that a subsequent orgasm can be achieved quickly.

Nuts, slang for testicles.

Orgasm, the climax phase of the sexual response cycle, characterized by intense physical pleasure, involuntary contractions of the lower pelvic and other muscles, and a general euphoric sensation.

Orgy, a group sex party which may include frequent rotation of sex partners, multiple simultaneous sex partners (gangbang), or may be limited to multiple couples.

P-Spot (Prostate Spot), a male erogenous zone inside the rectum where pressure can be applied to the prostate gland.

Package, slang for penis, or sometimes for vagina.

Paraurethral Gland, a gland of prostatic tissue corresponding to the prostate in men. It is a female erogenous zone located just above and on either side of the urethral opening, and it may be a source of fluid in female ejaculations.

Pearl Necklace, slang for semen ejaculated onto a woman's chest.

Penis, the male sexual organ for penetrating a woman's vagina and depositing sperm.

Petting, stroking, brushing, massaging, or caressing your spouse. Heavy petting involves touching the genitals.

Plug, slang for intercourse and the name of a sex toy that is inserted into the anus.

Pornography (Porn), sexually explicit media of any kind (writing, video, picture, video game, sculpture, etc).

Pocket Pussy, a sex toy, an artificial vagina used for male masturbation.

Popping a Cherry, a man having sex with a virgin woman.

Pound/Pounding, slang for deep vaginal intercourse where the tip of the penis touches the posterior fornix, near the back of the vagina.

Prick, slang for penis.

Pussy, slang for vagina.

Quickie, slang for having sex with the goal of at least one spouse reaching orgasm as quickly as possible.

Rack, slang for breasts.

Reaming, slang for anal intercourse.

Rimming, slang for using one person's tongue on another person's anus (very dangerous to health).

Rocks, slang for testicles.

Screw/Screwing, slang for vaginal or anal intercourse.

Sadomasochism (S&M), the abnormal creation of sexual arousal from inflicting pain or humiliation on one's self or on another person.

Scrotum, a sack of skin hanging below the penis which contains the testicles.

Semen, a male fluid containing sperm and seminal plasma produced by secretions of the seminal vesicle, prostate, and bulbourethral glands. Excreted through the penis in the process of ejaculation.

Sexually Transmitted Disease (STD), an infection transmitted between people by vaginal or anal intercourse, or by oral sex.

Shag, British slang for vaginal intercourse.

Shaft, slang for penis.

Skene's Gland, another term for paraurethral gland.

Spooge, slang for semen.

Soft-core, another word for erotica.

Spreading, slang for a woman seductively spreading her legs (clothed or unclothed) or her labia (unclothed).

Spunk, slang for semen.

STD, Sexually Transmitted Disease.

Strap-On, a sex toy, an artificial penis with harness. Worn by a wife to penetrate her husband's anus and pretend she's the man and he's the woman, or worn by a husband to penetrate his wife's vagina and anus at the same time.

Stripping, removing one's clothes in front of their spouse in as seductive a manner as possible.

Suck/Sucking, slang for fellatio, or less commonly for cunnilingus or sucking on a breast.

Sucking Cock, slang for fellatio.

Sucking Off, slang for fellatio, or particularly for fellatio that results in the husband ejaculating in his wife's mouth and her swallowing his semen.

Swapping, slang for married couples exchanging spouses for sexual activities.

Swinging, slang for frequently changing sex partners among married couples.

Sybian, a saddle-mounted dildo and vibrator combination.

Tail, slang for anus, buttocks, or vagina. Also a sex toy resembling an animal tail that attaches to a waist belt or a butt plug.

Tantric Sex, an ancient Indian spiritual tradition with a goal of eliminating orgasm from sexual intercourse in order to increase enjoyment of the pre-orgasmic states.

Tent Pole, slang for erect penis.

Testicles, two glandular organs in the male scrotum which produce both sperm (spermatozoa) and male sex hormones such as testosterone.

Tit Job, slang for mammary intercourse.

Tits, slang for breasts.

Titties, slang for breasts.

Tool, slang for penis.

Tongue Fucking, the husband or wife inserting their tongue into their spouses mouth (French kiss) or their ear, simulating vaginal intercourse, or the husband inserting his tongue into his wife's vagina.

Turn-Off, anything that quenches sexual arousal.

Turn-On, anything that causes sexual arousal.

U-Spot, another term for the para-urethral gland.

Wet Dream, an erotic dream that results in an ejaculation.

Wet Socks, slang for extreme arousal, implying that vaginal lubrication or pre-ejaculatory fluid has run all the way down the legs to the socks.

Vagina, a muscular tube with an external opening in a woman's pelvic region, below the clitoris and above the anus, and leading to the uterus. The vagina receives the penis during vaginal intercourse.

Vaginal Tenting, a slight increase in the length and width of vagina during sex, coinciding with the uterus rising slightly.

Venereal Disease, obsolete name for sexually transmitted diseases (STD's).

Vibrator, a sex toy, a mechanical device that creates vibrations and is either held against erogenous zones of the body or inserted into the vagina or anus in order to stimulate nerves for sexual arousal.

Virgin, a man or woman who has never had sex with another person.

INDEX

A

Ability, 16, 23, 30, 36, 55, 76,
147, 148, 156, 169, 177, 180,
182, 183, 184, 192
Abnormal, i, 43, 44, 84, 87,
117, 278
Abnormal Sex, i, 84
Abortion, i, 20, 33, 74, 78, 79,
80
Abstinence, 45, 75, 89
Abuse, 8, 130, 174, 177
Acceptability, 26, 98, 99, 101,
103, 106, 121, **124**, 186, 192,
301
Acclimation, iii, 183, 184, 185,
187, 188
Acclimation Phrases, 184, 185
Acquaintance, 111, 249
Actions, 21, 102, 140, 163, 171,
184, 189, 194, 231
Activities, 14, 36, 40, 41, 47,
48, 50, 81, 83, 84, 86, 87,
88, 92, 93, 104, 108, 112,
116, 117, 118, 120, 149, 156,
160, 167, 174, 178, 179, 181,
199, 204, 205, 239, 273,
275, 279
Addiction, 84, 87, 88, 120, 251
Adoption, 20, 78, 79
Adult, 17, 20, 95, 106, 117, 118,
121, 122, 150, 156, 162, 172,
179, 192, 194, 237
Adulterous Fantasy, 196, 201
Adultery, 82, 84, 96, 97, 108,
114, 127, 130, 180, 196, 200,
201, 273
Advantages, ii, 34, 38, 72, 80,
91, 107, 113, 116, 120, 123,
137, 150, 161, 166, 187, 192,
219, 228, 253
Age, 1, 9, 10, 14, 26, 82, 109,
110, 129, 169, 205, 206,
207, 257, 263, 301
Agreement, 25, 30, 52, 71, 81,
83, 92, 94, 128, 137, 150,
153, 156, 199, 200, 221, 223,
229, 231, 240, 250
Alternative Sex, ii, 147, 169,
170
Alternatives, ii, 16, 36, 137,
147, 156, 157, 169, 170
Anal Intercourse, i, 33, 54, 55,
112, 273, 274, 276, 277, 278,
279
Anatomy, i, 33, 34, 43, 184,
189
Female, i, 33, 34
Male, i, 33, 43
Anger, 21, 31, 50, 80, 110, 137,
177, 186, 240
Animals, 81, 82, 95, 98, 106,
131, 147, 181, 215, 226, 264,
265, 279
Animation, 107
Anticipation, 51, 148, 168
Anus, 34, 35, 36, 39, 41, 43, 46,
48, 51, 54, 55, 65, 77, 139,
140, 142, 144, 145, 159, 162,
185, 197, 232, 273, 274, 275,
277, 278, 279, 280
Anxiety, 57, 80, 140, 149, 150,
170, 174, 177, 184, 188, 263
Appeal, iii, 26, 179, 181
Approval, 83, 113, 128, 131,
143, 153, 215
Areola, 39, 41
Armpit Intercourse, 56
A-Spot, 39, 56, 185, 273
Assertiveness, 12, 52, 93, 148
Attractive, 35, 267, 277
Attractiveness, 26
Audio, 107, 114, 139, 192
Awareness, 40, 41, 47, 48, 112,
228

B

Babies, 1, 2, 20, 70, 71, 73, 78,
79, 80, 91, 114, 131, 135, 147,
149, 165, 166, 167, 168, 179,
190, 213

INDEX

INDEX

INDEX

INDEX

Force, 22, 24, 57, 58, 83, 251, 266
Forced-Sex Fantasy, 196, 202
Foreplay, i, 15, 33, 50, 51, 93, 147, 153, 156, 163, 174, 185, 207, 275
Foreskin, 43
Fornication, 108, 275
Fornix, 34, 273, 278
French Kissing, 41, 48, 185, 275, 280
Frenulum, 45, 46, 48, 162
Frequency, 125, 159, 193, 205, 209, 211
Friends, 7, 15, 16, 23, 24, 83, 168, 177, 219, 221, 223, 234, 236, 240, 242, 243, 245, 248, 249, 251, 271, 275
Friendships, 23, 243, 245, 263
Fright, 110, 177, 259
Front-To-Back, 59
Fun, 8, 22, 23, 30, 69, 91, 151, 165, 166, 180, 196, 197, 199, 203, 204, 245, 247, 260

G

Gag Reflex, 161, 162
Games, 107, 192, 194
Garage, 139, 182
Gardasil, 19
Gender, iii, 55, 65, 112, 195, 196, 197, 215, 268
Gender-Reversal Fantasy, iii, 55, 65, 112, 195, 196, 197, 215, 268
Genitals, 3, 34, 35, 40, 41, 43, 47, 48, 51, 53, 63, 87, 107, 123, 127, 138, 150, 275, 277, 278
Gifts, 5, 12, 25, 83, 134, 139, 143, 174, 180, 198, 271, 277
Girl, 2, 10, 18, 19, 21, 22, 127, 153, 219, 228, 235, 237, 254, 256, 260
Girlfriend, 218
Glans (Penis Glans), 45, 46, 48, 162
Gloves, 43, 51, 220, 232
Goblet, 52, 53
God, ii, 5, 11, 18, 28, 71, 83, 90, 94, 95, 98, 100, 106, 114, 115, 116, 124, 125, 128, 129, 130, 131, 133, 134, 136, 137, 138, 139, 155, 183, 195, 201, 216, 271, 272, 301
Godly Sex, ii, 92
Granddaughter, 1, 2, 9, 11, 174, 301
Grandma
    Anne, 1, 8, 44, 81, 129, 131, 181, 199, 301
    Brenda, 8, 56, 58, 181, 199
    Caroline, 2, 3, 4, 8, 51, 155, 181, 195
    Dora, 8, 53, 107, 125, 133
    Elizabeth, 3, 4, 8, 57, 82, 104, 107, 110, 111, 112, 144, 181
    Grandma Flora, 3, 4, 7, 9, 11, 131, 134, 199
    Grandma Victoria, 9, 171, 174
    Great-Grandma Nora, 9
    Great-Great-Grandma Theodora, 9
    Heather, 9, 121, 181, 205, 206, 207, 208, 209, 210, 211
    Jennifer, 9, 21, 107, 118, 152, 181
    Kelly, 9, 160, 181
    Lily, 4, 10
    Rachael, 4, 10, 181, 196, 240
    Synthia, 10, 20, 39, 46, 50, 53, 71, 74, 113, 118, 119, 121, 124, 131, 137, 156, 159, 175, 180, 215
    Yvette, 10, 54, 112, 181
Grandma's Ooo-aah Club, 192
Grandmother, 1, 3, 243, 263, 301
Gratification, 96
Greek, 8, 88, 96, 100, 115, 237
Groom, 30, 113, 234, 251, 267
Group Sex, 110, 111, 202, 277
Group-Sex Fantasy, 196, 202
G-Spot, 34, 36, 39, 185, 275
Guides, ii, iii, **124**, 132, 140, 141, 147, 152, 164, 183, 187, 188, 271, 272, 301
Guilt, 27, 80, 108, 116, 120, 124, 125, 132, 133, 140
Gynecologist, 31, 70, 231

H

M

N

INDEX

INDEX

INDEX

INDEX

INDEX

INDEX

INDEX

ForeWord Clarion Review, by Jeannine Chartier Hanscom:

For author Anne Wright (writing under a pseudonym), sharing sex advice among the women in her family has become a tradition, a coming-of-age ritual passed down from grandmother to granddaughter for at least eight generations. *Grandma's Sex Handbook* is a compilation of that very candid and explicit advice about sex, meant to be passed along to an engaged and presumably inexperienced woman prior to her wedding night.

"Grandma's sex advice is based on helping Christian women who really want to treat their husbands as well as they can physically and emotionally, and maximize the joy in their own lives based on relationships that are strong and healthy," the author writes.

The "Grandma" of the title is actually a conglomeration of several women in Wright's family. The book encourages women to accept and embrace their sexuality as God's natural design. As Wright puts it, "There is a sinful nature that Godly people should resist, but a normal sex drive is *not* part of a sinful nature, it is part of God's design...God gave us sex, and he gave us libidos that periodically demand sexual satisfaction."

Grandma's Sex Handbook is well organized and extremely thorough, written in a conversational tone that puts readers at ease. The author makes it clear that the intended audience consists primarily of married or soon to be married Christian women. While recognizing that not every reader will feel immediately comfortable with the subject matter, as "It's common knowledge: most Christians struggle with sex," Wright nevertheless forges ahead with a forthright and honest exploration of nearly every aspect of sexuality between couples. She includes several personal stories, Bible references with subsequent exposition to support conclusions, and advice for couples with physical limitations due to partial paralysis or health concerns. However, the author does not shy away from candid discussion of pregnancy, STDs, the acceptability of sex toys and fantasy within a marriage, and more unusual sexual practices. A comprehensive index, a "Glossary of Sexual Terms," and a "Sex Fantasy Cookbook" with more than 100 fantasy scenarios is also included.

Wright's statement in the foreword that the book is of an "explicit nature" is not an overstatement. Readers should be aware that in addition to the frank language, the book includes several graphic photos and very detailed drawings as well as sections that deal with what the author terms "Wild Sex," all of which more conservative readers may find distasteful.

Grandma's Sex Handbook is written with a simplicity that illuminates rather than condescends, yet the extremely explicit nature is such that it may miss its target audience of young Christian women. For those readers who remain undaunted by the very direct, "anything goes" approach to discussing sexuality, however, the book could prove helpful and enlightening.

www.ingramcontent.com/pod-product-compliance
Lightning Source LLC
LaVergne TN
LVHW051455080426
835509LV00017B/1771